Implantable Cardioverter Defibrillator Stored ECGs

Luc J. Jordaens and Dominic A.M.J. Theuns

Implantable Cardioverter Defibrillator Stored ECGs

Clinical Management and Case Reports

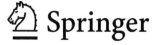 Springer

Luc J. Jordaens, MD, PhD
Erasmus Medical
Centre Rotterdam,
The Netherlands

Dominic A.M.J. Theuns, PhD
Erasmus Medical
Centre Rotterdam,
The Netherlands

British Library Cataloguing in Publication Data
Jordaens, L. (Luc)
    Implantable cardioverter defibrillator stored ECGS :
    Clinical management and case reports
    1. Implantable cardioverter-defibrillators
    2. Electrocardiography
    I. Title II. Theuns, Dominic A. M. J.
    617. 4'12'0645
ISBN-13: 978-1-84628-679-7

Library of Congress Control Number: 2006939780

ISBN 978-1-84628-679-7   e-ISBN 978-1-84628-680-3

Printed on acid-free paper

9 8 7 6 5 4 3 2 1

Springer Science+Business Media
springer.com

Contents

Foreword

In recent years there has been a tremendous increase in ICD use for primary and secondary prevention of life-threatening ventricular arrhythmias, and nowadays many of our patients are equipped with such a device.

Unfortunately, understanding of how the ICD functions and how to recognize appropriate and inappropriate interventions by the device, remains terra incognita for most cardiologists.

This book is therefore very welcome. The authors have succeeded in providing us with a well written manual on how to get information about the way the device interprets an arrhythmia or pseudo arrhythmia and which action is taken by the device thereafter.

Inappropriate ICD shocks are (unfortunately) still common. They can lead to anxiety and depression. The ability to recognize those events, to identify their cause, and to take the appropriate steps to correct and prevent them, is essential for the health professional active in the ICD area.

Currently, different devices from different companies are being used with adaptations and increasing sophistication in the newer models. The authors point out that a systematic approach to the analysis of the device function is essential. How to do this is illustrated in the many examples given, going from older devices to the most recent ones.

ICD use will increase, for example in relation with resynchronization therapy in the heart failure patient. Remote interpretation and programming of the ICD will become possible in the near future.

All these developments make the educational material, which is so well presented in this book, not only of value for the health professional actively involved in the implantable cardiac device area, but is also recommended for any cardiologist who takes care of an ICD patient.

Hein J. Wellens
Emeritus Professor of Cardiology
University of Maastricht
The Netherlands

Preface

Implantable cardioverter-defibrillator (ICD) therapy is one of the most important advances in the therapeutic approach of cardiovascular patients, with a life saving benefit exceeding that of all antiarrhythmic drugs. Since the first defibrillator implantation in 1980, the technology, diagnostic and therapeutic options have dramatically evolved, widening the indication area from secondary to primary prevention of sudden cardiac death. Over the intervening 25 years, implantable defibrillator therapy has become first line therapy for patients who survived cardiac arrest and for patients who are at risk for life-threatening ventricular arrhythmias. Its combination with cardiac resynchronisation therapy proved to be a major asset for heart failure patients, for whom now a real arrhythmia and heart failure management device became available. On the other hand, randomised trials have shown that huge numbers of patients might benefit from prophylactic treatment with simple ICD's.

The implantation rate in Europe is finally increasing but still not at the level of the U.S.A. Anyhow, ICD's are now considered as a part of regular health care, and physicians and personnel at coronary care units, emergency departments and general wards will often encounter patients who have an ICD, or who received an ICD shock or who were symptomatic.

A wide variety of cardiologists, electrophysiologists, fellows, anesthesiologists, nurses, and cardiovascular technicians are involved in delivering care to ICD patients. In addition to the diverse background of these individuals caring for ICD patients, defibrillator therapy became more complex over the last two decades. The advances in technology resulted in the development of tiered-therapy devices, physiologic pacing, resynchronization therapy, extended diagnostic functions, advanced arrhythmia discrimination, stored electrograms and the possibility to telemeter and transmit the data in the device over the internet or over the GSM network.

Device implantation is a fairly common intervention, the difficulties of understanding events during follow-up remain huge, at least for the untrained individual. Training is often given by the device company, and seldom covers the clinical needs, and the advances of devices from other companies.

In order to meet the needs of physicians, scientists, nurses, and cardiovascular technicians, a book that covers this subject in a comprehensive fashion is necessary. The purpose of this textbook is to present information on device diagnostics and clinical cases that we encountered in our daily practice, and to share our experience with all who would like to know more of this advanced electrocardiography.

Rotterdam, January 2007

DAMJ Theuns   LJ Jordaens

Acknowledgements

This book would have been impossible without the support of many people in our hospital and elsewhere. We would like to mention all cardiologists of our department, and especially those who are or have been active in the EP group: Geert Kimman, Tamas Szili-Torok, Peter Klootwijk, Marcoen Scholten, Jan Res, Andrew Thornton, Joris Mekel, Maximo Rivero-Ayerza, Yves van Belle, and Emile Jessurun.

The effort of the technicians of our group who collected many interesting electrograms has to be greatly appreciated (Ronald van der Perk, Roel de Ruiter, Max Miltenburg, Paul Knops, Ronald Luijten, and Wout de Ruiter). The entire EP team was very supportive, while we were gathering additional data... Also to be gratefully acknowledged is Grant Weston of Springer, who understood that this book merited an important place in this series.

Further we would like to dedicate this book to Maria, Lauren, Fien and Floor . Maybe they will once understand why their fathers had so much fun while they were working on the PC.

1
Diagnostics and Therapy by the ICD: Better than the Cardiologist?

From the time of introduction of the Implantable Cardioverter Defibrillator (ICD), the device has evolved from a simple shock-box to a complete arrhythmia management device. Diagnostics or interpretation of what the defibrillator had done with the patient and his arrhythmias has always been a matter of concern for the cardiologist [1]. In the beginning, the non-programmable devices were limited to shock delivery, and it was only possible to assess the charge time and to read the number of delivered shocks (Figure 1.1).

Advances in diagnostic information have paralleled the improvements in arrhythmia treatment (pacing, antitachycardia pacing, atrioversion). The current generation of ICDs offers an array of diagnostic information, including stored electrograms. Analysis of this diagnostic information has not only improved the management of patients, but also contributed to an increased understanding of triggers precipitating device therapy. It becomes evident that the amount of data available in a device will be extremely helpful to the experienced cardiologist to understand the arrhythmia, the involved mechanism, and the underlying disease. Physiological information derived from measurements like thoracic impedance, lead tension, and oxygen saturation will become available and will even change our management of heart failure patients. It is clear that device information has to be reliable; therefore it has to be studied, understood, and often corrected. Cardiologists should not solely rely on information as provided by the manufacturer, but be prepared to teach other physicians (who are not electrophysiologists), nurses, and technicians. They should be able to engage in a discussion with the industry at a high level. We hope that this book will be a contribution to be successful in this area.

Historical Perspective of Diagnostic Information in ICDs

In the first-generation devices, the definition of "appropriate" therapy relied on the clinical history of the patient, the presence or absence of hemodynamically significant symptoms, or concomitant ECG monitoring. Diagnostic information remained limited after the introduction of programmable devices (Figure 1.2).

1

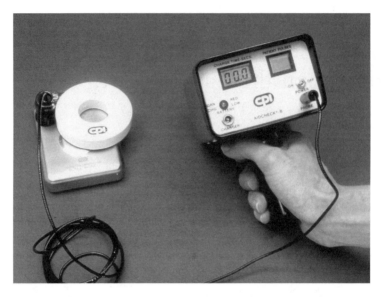

Figure 1.1. Read-out of the device, using a doughnut-magnet, which allowed capacitor reformation. Via audible tones synchronicity with the R-wave was assessed (AID and AICD, Intec; later Ventak 1500 series, CPI).

The second-generation ICDs had recording of numerical RR intervals, often tabular, sometimes with device activity markers. This storage allowed analysis of the rate of the arrhythmia preceding and following ICD therapy. Differentiation of arrhythmias was based on the regularity of RR intervals. Irregular RR intervals suggested atrial fibrillation (AF), while regular RR intervals could indicate sinus tachycardia, arial flutter, or atrial tachycardia as well as ventricular tachycardia (Figure 1.3).

Appropriate ICD therapy for ventricular arrhythmias without hemodynamically significant symptoms was soon demonstrated in patients [2, 3]. With third-generation devices, the most significant advance in diagnostic information was the storage of intracardiac electrogram recordings (Figure 1.4). This diagnostic information included recording of RR intervals preceding and following the arrhythmia, and stored electrograms with real-time marker channels of arrhythmias triggering ICD therapy. It became clear that this bit of information would be helpful in the interpretation of clinical data.

The Diagnosis of Ventricular Tachycardia: A Continuing Story with a Happy End?

The manifestation of a regular broad complex tachycardia on the electrocardiogram can be due to ventricular tachycardia or supraventricular tachycardia with aberrant conduction. For the accurate differential diagnosis of a broad

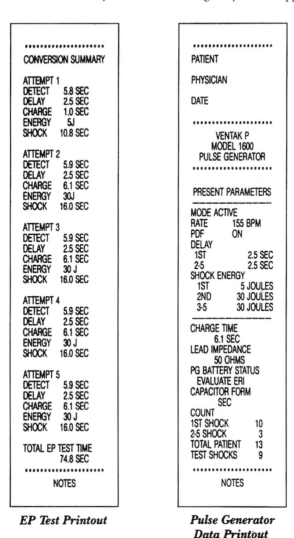

EP Test Printout

Pulse Generator Data Printout

FIGURE 1.2. EP test data and pulse generator data printouts of one of the first programmable ICDs (Ventak P 1600, Guidant).

complex tachycardia, several famous cardiologists have developed diagnostic algorithms [4–6]. Most of these diagnostic algorithms are based on features of the QRS complex, including QRS width, morphology in the precordial leads and axis in the frontal plane, and features of atrioventricular dissociation like the presence of P waves independent of QRS complexes, fusion, or capture beats. The diagnostic algorithms implement these features into a step-by-step diagnostic hierarchy. Despite these algorithms, misdiagnoses are still common [6]. A major limitation of these diagnostic algorithms is imperfect

```
LAST EPISODE DETECTION SEQUENCE:
-19. R-R INTERVAL- 470 MS
-18. R-R INTERVAL- 370 MS
-17. R-R INTERVAL- 280 MS
-16. R-R INTERVAL- 280 MS
-15. R-R INTERVAL- 250 MS
-14. R-R INTERVAL- 280 MS
-13. R-R INTERVAL- 280 MS
-12. R-R INTERVAL- 270 MS
-11. R-R INTERVAL- 270 MS
-10. R-R INTERVAL- 290 MS
 -9. R-R INTERVAL- 290 MS
 -8. R-R INTERVAL- 280 MS
 -7. R-R INTERVAL- 300 MS
 -6. R-R INTERVAL- 280 MS
 -5. R-R INTERVAL- 290 MS
 -4. R-R INTERVAL- 290 MS
 -3. R-R INTERVAL- 300 MS
 -2. R-R INTERVAL- 290 MS
 -1. R-R INTERVAL- 270 MS
 -0. R-R INTERVAL- 300 MS
 -0. VF DETECTED
```

FIGURE 1.3. Interval table (Medtronic PCD 7219). After a rather long interval of 470 ms, and a much shorter coupling of 370 ms, a more or less regular tachycardia becomes present with cycle length of 250 to 300 ms. After these intervals the device reports that ventricular fibrillation (VF) was detected.

ascertainment of electrocardiogram features. It is thought that devices with accurate atrial information will be extremely helpful.

Stored electrograms have increased our understanding of events leading to ventricular tachycardia, ventricular fibrillation, or sudden death, also in exceptional occasions or syndromes [7–14]. In this book, we will try to draw the attention of the reader also to these features.

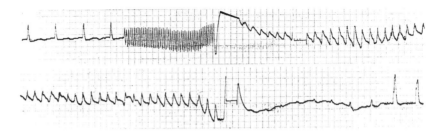

FIGURE 1.4. Electrogram recorded via wand and ECG machine (Guidant, Ventak 1625). With alternating current, a polymorphic wide QRS arrhythmia is induced with smaller amplitude than the preceding rhythm. After a shock (lower strip, upward spike) the amplifier is saturated, initially resulting in lower amplitudes of restored normal sinus rhythm.

References

1. Mirowski M, Mower MM, Reid PR, Watkins L, Langer A. The automatic implantable defibrillator. New modality for treatment of life-threatening ventricular arrhythmias. Pacing Clin Electrophysiol 1982;5:384-401.
2. Fogoros RN, Elson JJ, Bonnet CA. Actuarial incidence and pattern of occurrence of shocks following implantation of the automatic implantable cardioverter defibrillator. Pacing Clin Electrophysiol 1989;12:1465-1473.
3. Maloney J, Masterson M, Khoury D, Trohman R, Wilkoff B, Simmons T, Morant V, Castle L. Clinical performance of the implantable cardioverter defibrillator: electrocardiographic documentation of 101 spontaneous discharges. Pacing Clin Electrophysiol 1991;14:280-285.
4. Wellens HJ, Bar FW, Lie KI. The value of the electrocardiogram in the differential diagnosis of a tachycardia with a widened QRS complex. Am J Med 1978;64:27-33.
5. Brugada P, Brugada J, Mont L, et al. A new approach to the differential diagnosis of a regular tachycardia with a wide QRS complex. Circulation 1991;83:1649-1659.
6. Griffith MJ, Garratt CJ, Mounsey P, et al. Ventricular tachycardia as default diagnosis in broad complex tachycardia. Lancet 1994;343:386-388.
7. Hook BG, Marchlinski FE. Value of ventricular electrogram recordings in the diagnosis of arrhythmias precipitating electrical device shock therapy. J Am Coll Cardiol 1991;17:989-990.
8. Marchlinski FE, Gottlieb CD, Sarter B, Finkle J, Hook B, Callans D, Schwartzman D. ICD data storage: Value in arrhythmia management. Pacing Clin Electrophysiol 1993;16:527-534.
9. Roelke M, Garan H, McGovern BA, Ruskin JN. Analysis of the initiation of spontaneous monomorphic ventricular tachycardia by stored intracardiac electrograms. J Am Coll Cardiol 1994;23:117-122.
10. Pratt CM, Greenway PS, Schoenfeld MH, Hibben ML, Reiffel JA. Exploration of the precision of classifying sudden cardiac death. Implications for the interpretation of clinical trials. Circulation 1996;93:519-524.
11. Meyerfeldt U, Schirdewan A, Wiedemann M, Schutt H, Zimmerman F, Luft FC, Dietz R. The mode of onset of ventricular tachycardia. A patient-specific phenomenon. Eur Heart J 1997;18:1956-1965.
12. Taylor E, Berger R, Hummel JD, Dinerman JL, Kenknight B, Arria AM, Tomaselli G, Calkins H. Analysis of the pattern of initiation of sustained ventricular arrhythmias in patients with implantable defibrillators. J Cardiovasc Electrophysiol 2000;11:719-726.
13. Kakishita M, Kurita T, Matsuo K, Taguchi A, Suyama K, Shimizu W, Aihara N, Kamakura S, Yamamoto F, Kobayashi J, Kosakai Y, Ohe T. Mode of onset of ventricular fibrillation in patients with Brugada syndrome detected by implantable cardioverter defibrillator therapy. J Am Coll Cardiol 2000;36:1646-1653.
14. Schimpf R, Wolpert C, Bianchi F, Giustetto C, Gaita F, Bauersfeld U, Borggrefe M. Congenital short QT syndrome and implantable cardioverter defibrillator treatment: inherent risk for inappropriate shock delivery. J Cardiovasc Electrophysiol 2003;14:1273-1277.

2
Rhythm Classification by Arrhythmia Management Devices

Summary

A reliable ICD needs both sensing of the endocardial signal and detection algorithms for arrhythmia diagnosis. Initially, the only target was ventricular fibrillation, but with the possibility of rate detection ventricular tachycardia could be detected as well. This led to the development of tiered-therapy devices with arrhythmia zones. Simple arrhythmia discriminators as stability and sudden onset became available, and proved to be very useful. The place of more complex algorithms is still unclear.

The ability of an ICD to reliably detect life-threatening ventricular arrhythmias is one of the most essential features of a device. It involves both sensing of the endocardial signal and the application of detection algorithms for arrhythmia diagnosis [1, 2]. The ICD must consistently sense all ventricular depolarizations to accurately determine the heart rate during sinus rhythm and tachyarrhythmias (Figure 2.1). The challenge is to reliably sense low amplitude signals during ventricular fibrillation and to avoid sensing of T waves or extracardiac signals (Figure 2.2).

Actually, two different endocardiac lead designs for sensing, either dedicated bipolar or integrated bipolar, are used. Bipolar epicardiac signals are only exceptionally necessary (pediatric patients, congenital heart disease) and pose specific problems (Figure 2.3). Sensing with a dedicated endocardiac bipolar system is accomplished between the tip electrode and a second ring electrode, approximately 10 mm from the tip. With the integrated bipolar configuration, sensing is accomplished between the tip electrode and the right ventricular shocking coil. Both dedicated and integrated bipolar lead sensing concepts are effective for sensing low amplitude signals during ventricular fibrillation.

Other sensing configurations have been used in different conditions or for specific devices, as a unipolar lead with a patch, or a can. Sensing of the left ventricular signal is now introduced for biventricular approaches (resynchronization).

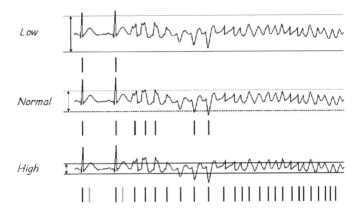

FIGURE 2.1. Different levels of sensitivity result in recognition (black vertical bars) of only the normal complexes (low sensitivity); recognition of normal complexes and ventricular premature beats (normal sensitivity); recognition of normal complexes, ventricular premature beats, and ventricular fibrillation (high sensitivity). The drawback in the last situation is that T-waves are sensed as well (grey bars).

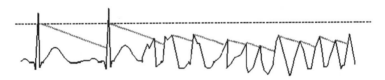

FIGURE 2.2. Current ICDs utilize either automatic gain control or auto-adjusting threshold to ensure reliable sensing. In automatic gain control, the sensing threshold is fixed while continuous adjustment of the gain is performed to ensure maximum sensing. With this method, the gain is increased when the amplitudes of the R wave decrease from large to small. In auto-adjusting threshold, the gain is fixed and the threshold is adjusted. Auto-adjusting threshold uses a constant amplification of the amplitude of the R wave, which becomes the starting amplitude of the time-decay threshold. The figure shows how the ventricular arrhythmia is correctly recognised because the threshold (dotted line) is adjusted after the QRS complexes, while the T-wave is not sensed.

Verification of Signals During Implantation

The lead electrogram and markers should be checked during implantation for evidence of correct sensing. Loose connections and oversensing of intracardiac or extracardiac signals should be recognized in this stage (Figure 2.4). If the patient had a previously implanted or abandoned ventricular lead in place, it is important to check for mechanical lead 'chatter' that can generate signals mimicking ventricular tachyarrhythmias. If lead 'chatter' is observed on the electrograms, a reposition of the lead is necessary. It seems wise to remove redundant leads. Connectors and adaptors are predisposed to additional noise, and should be avoided.

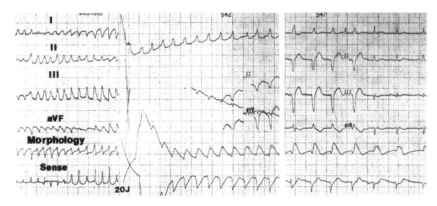

FIGURE 2.3. Ventricular fibrillation with conversion to sinus rhythm after a short irregular episode with wide QRS complexes (ventricular wide band and bipolar electrograms are displayed). The first electrogram is taken between epicardiac patches and shows impressive ST segment elevation, also after normalisation of the QRS width. This will certainly affect sensing properties directly after a shock.

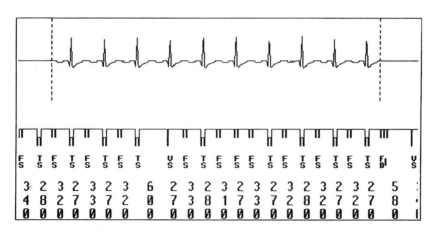

FIGURE 2.4. Regular sinus rhythm (ventricular bipolar electrogram). It is interpreted as tachycardia intervals (TS), alternating with fibrillatory intervals (FS), except at one interval of 600 ms. This phenomenon is due to sensing of the T wave. This error finally leads to detection of fibrillation (FD).

Early Devices: Detection of Ventricular Fibrillation

The original detection algorithm in the automatic implantable defibrillator (AID^{TM}) was the probability density function (PDF), conceived to detect sinusoidal rhythms (Intec Systems) [3]. The PDF processed the electrical signal to define the proportion of the cardiac cycle that this signal was deviating from the baseline (Figure 2.5).

The algorithm was based on the observation that the signal during ventricular fibrillation spends the majority of its time away from the isoelectric

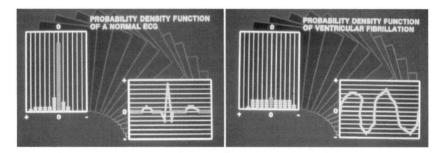

FIGURE 2.5. Probability density function (modified, from Intec) during sinus rhythm (left) and ventricular fibrillation (right).

baseline as compared to the signal during sinus rhythm. CPI shortly proposed a so-called 'turning point morphology' criterion (TPM), derived from the electrogram recorded between the shock leads. The principle was that electrograms with a certain percentage of isoelectric time and a high slew rate would not satisfy the TPM criteria. It was felt that these morphology criteria postponed intervention [4].

Rate-only Detection

The basic goal of the ICD is to detect and subsequently terminate life-threatening ventricular tachyarrhythmias. The most fundamental criterion for the detection of ventricular tachyarrhythmias is based on rate. This is measured by assessing the duration of the cardiac cycle length (time divided by rate) on a beat-to-beat basis. Each detected ventricular interval is compared with the programmed detection zones. This basic detection algorithm measures and counts ventricular intervals to detect a tachyarrhythmia if it fulfils the criteria of ventricular rate over a certain, predefined duration. With correct sensing, this method ensures 100% sensitivity of ventricular tachyarrhythmias with rates above the programmed detection rate. However, rate-only detection has a poor specificity in arrhythmia discrimination. The reported incidence of inappropriate therapy ranged between 16 and 41% [5–8]. This incidence may have been underestimated due to the lack of electrogram storage. The definition of 'appropriate' therapy relied on concomitant ECG monitoring. The fact that atrial tachyarrhythmias contributed to the incidence of inappropriate therapy was established.

With tiered-therapy devices (providing antitachycardia pacing for slower tachycardias), the inappropriate detection of atrial tachyarrhythmias became a greater problem [9]. This is due to the increased probability of rate overlap between the target ventricular tachyarrhythmias and atrial tachyarrhythmias, as lower detection zones can be programmed.

Detection Zones

In modern ICDs, the range of ventricular rates is divided into a bradyarrhythmia, a normal, and up to three tachyarrhythmia detection zones (Figure 2.6). In all ICDs, the highest detection zone is called the 'fibrillation' zone. In order for a tachyarrhythmia to be detected and assigned to a given detection zone, it must exhibit a certain number of intervals (duration). For this duration criterion different methods of counting are used (consecutive interval counting, probabilistic counting, or a combination of these).

Probabilistic counting algorithms are used for the detection of *ventricular fibrillation*. This algorithm requires a defined proportion of ventricular intervals within a sliding window to be shorter than the programmed detection interval for fibrillation (X of Y counter). This method reduces the chance of underdetection of ventricular fibrillation due to the irregularity of ventricular intervals and the continuously changing amplitude of the signal. In Medtronic ICDs, for example, 75% of consecutive intervals must be within the fibrillation detection zone. In the Guidant algorithm, a fixed window width of 10 intervals is used. Initially, 8 of 10 intervals are required within the fibrillation detection zone for rate detection to be met, and at least 6 of 10 intervals must remain in the detection zone for a programmed detection time.

The counting algorithm for *ventricular tachycardia* may be either probabilistic or consecutive in design. The consecutive-interval algorithm diminishes the risk of inappropriate therapy for atrial fibrillation, without compromising the sensitivity for detection of ventricular tachycardias. In consecutive-interval algorithms, the counter increments every time when an interval is measured within the detection zone. An interval outside the detection zone will reset the counter to zero. For patients with both slow and fast ventricular tachycardias, the programming of two tachycardia detection zones allow zone-specific detection and therapies. The programming of slow tachycardia detection zones increases the risk of inappropriate therapies for atrial tachyarrhythmias [9, 10].

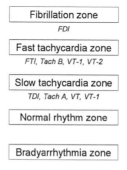

Figure 2.6. Detection and therapy zones. The detection and assignment of ventricular tachyarrhythmias into a specific zone is dependent on the programming of the range of ventricular rates into non-overlapping zones. Abbreviations: FDI = fibrillation detection interval; FTI = fast tachycardia interval; TDI = tachycardia detection interval; Tach A, VT, or VT-1 = slower tachycardia limit; Tach B, VT-1, or VT-2 = faster tachycardia limit.

Interval-based Discriminators

One of the most important limitations of ICD detection is inappropriate therapy delivered for atrial tachyarrhythmias. Interval-based discriminators as 'sudden onset' and 'stability' were developed to improve the specificity of arrhythmia discrimination [11–13].

The discriminator 'sudden onset' aims at distinguishing sinus tachycardia (gradual onset) from VT (abrupt onset) (Figure 2.7). Sudden onset has a high specificity for rejecting sinus tachycardia [11, 13]. Despite this high specificity, this discriminator may cause underdetection of VT originating during atrial tachyarrhythmias and VT starting with a rate below the programmed detection rate [11]. The risk for underdetection of VT is increased with higher programmed values for 'sudden onset' [13].

The discriminator 'stability', or rate regularity, uses an interval variability threshold to differentiate VT characterized by stable intervals from atrial fibrillation with irregular ventricular response. Stability has proven to be reliable in the rejection of atrial fibrillation with a mean ventricular rate <170 min^{-1} [12, 14]. However, the performance of 'stability' is dependent on the rate of the ventricular response, as the degree of interval variability decreases at faster rates [14]. The reported incidence of inappropriate therapy ranged between 6 and 21% on a per-patient basis [15–17].

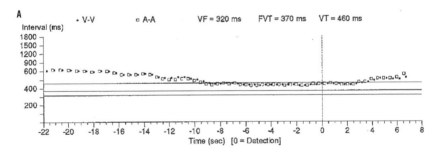

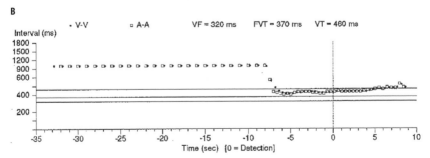

Figure 2.7. Panel A, interval plot showing a tachyarrhythmia with a gradual onset. Panel B, interval plot showing a tachyarrhythmia with a sudden onset. (Medtronic, model GEM 7271 DR). □ A-A: AA intervals; • V-V: VV intervals; FVT = fast ventricular tachycardia; VF = ventricular fibrillation; VT = ventricular tachycardia.

Initially, both discriminators have been used infrequently because physicians were concerned about underdetection of VTs. Serious underdetection was observed in only a minor proportion of the episodes.

The addition of a *safety timer* (duration) may prevent underdetection of VT. If a tachyarrhythmia satisfies the ventricular rate criterion and the discriminators indicate SVT, the safety timer will override the discriminators and therapy will be delivered. However, this feature ensured 100% sensitivity for VT but at the price of decreased specificity for rejection of SVT [18]. In a case control study, the interval-based discriminators 'sudden onset' and 'stability' reduce inappropriate therapies due to atrial fibrillation and sinus tachycardia [17]. The major limitation of 'sudden onset' and 'stability' is the inefficiency to reject sudden onset atrial tachyarrhythmias with a consistent atrioventricular (AV) relation, e.g. atrial tachycardia or atrial flutter. Complex algorithms with the addition of atrial information might improve the specificity of arrhythmia discrimination.

Dual-chamber Discrimination

An early plea for the addition of atrial sensing to improve arrhythmia discrimination was proposed by Furman as early as in 1982 [19]. The comparison between atrial and ventricular rates is a simple and effective arrhythmia discriminator. In the majority of VTs, the ventricular rate is faster than the atrial rate. Limitations of this simple criterion are the underdetection of VTs with 1:1 VA conduction and ventricular tachyarrhythmias during atrial fibrillation. To address this limitation, the analysis of the AV relationship was postulated as a feature of interest to discriminate sinus tachycardia from VT [20]. Measurement of the AV relationship provides a reliable diagnostic tool for AV association. Further, timing relationships between atrial and ventricular electrograms can be used to identify atrial tachyarrhythmias with stable AV conduction.

All dual-chamber algorithms comprise both single- and dual-chamber discriminators (Table 2.1). Dual-chamber discrimination algorithms include comparison of atrial and ventricular rates and/or measures of the AV relationship. The algorithms in dual-chamber devices can be roughly divided into two groups: (1) Comparison of atrial and ventricular rates (rate branches) and (2) Hierarchical analysis of the atrioventricular relationship.

Dual-chamber Algorithms Based on Analysis of the Atrioventricular Relationship

A hierarchical structure of single- and dual-chamber arrhythmia discrim-inators is applied in the algorithms PARAD, PARAD+ (ELA Medical), and PR Logic (Medtronic). The PARAD algorithm (P And R Based

TABLE 2.1. Arrhythmia discrimination components in dual-chamber algorithms.

	Biotronik	ELA Medical	Guidant	Medtronic	St. Jude Medical
Single-chamber detection					
Stability	+	+	+	+	+
Sudden onset	+	+	+		+
Sustained duration	+		+		+
Dual-chamber detection					
Atrial vs ventricular rates	+		+		+
AV association	+	+		+	+
Timing relationship	+			+	
Chamber of origin		+			

AV = atrioventricular

Arrhythmia Detection) first analyses the stability of the rhythm, then atrioventricular association, onset, and finally the chamber of origin (Figure 2.8) [21]. The chamber of origin is used to discriminate between ventricular tachyarrhythmias and atrial tachyarrhythmias with 1:1 AV relation by identification of atrial activity preceding ventricular activity or vice versa. In PARAD+, the additional criterion 'long cycle search' can be activated to inhibit therapy for atrial fibrillation with fast ventricular response.

The PR Logic algorithm (Figure 2.9) is based on the timing relationship of atrial activity with respect to ventricular activity. For atrioventricular relationship analysis, each RR interval is divided into four zones. Arrhythmia classification is based on PP and RR findings. An episode receives a code, which is compared with templates in a library of arrhythmias. PP intervals and

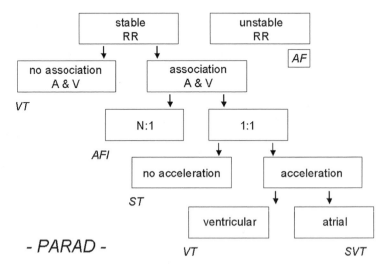

FIGURE 2.8. PARAD algorithm, as developed by ELA. AF: atrial fibrillation; AFI: atrial flutter; RR: RR intervals; ST: sinus tachycardia; SVT: supraventricular tachycardia; VT: ventricular tachycardia.

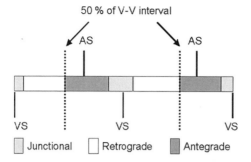

FIGURE 2.9. PR Logic algorithm as developed by Medtronic. The two cycles before the event are broken down into segments so that the result can be compared with a library of arrhythmias and a decision can be taken whether the arrhythmia is of ventricular origin.

AV relation are used for identification of atrial tachyarrhythmias. Stability of RR intervals and AV dissociation are used to identify ventricular arrhythmias when atrial fibrillation is present [22].

In both algorithms therapy is delivered unless a discriminator identifies an atrial tachyarrhythmia.

Dual-chamber Algorithms Based on Rate Branches

Comparison of atrial and ventricular rates is applied in several algorithms. The dual-chamber algorithms in Biotronik (Figure 2.10) and St. Jude Medical initially divide tachyarrhythmias into three rate branches: ventricular rate > atrial rate, ventricular rate < atrial rate, and ventricular rate = atrial rate. In the latter two branches, applicable single- and dual-chamber arrhythmia discriminators are applied to classifiy the arrhythmia [23]. In case of the ventricular rate = atrial rate branch, the onset criterion and analysis of the

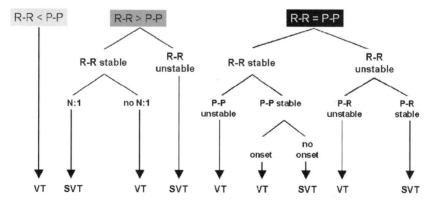

FIGURE 2.10. SMART algorithm (Biotronik), with three rate branches. PP: atrial intervals; RR: ventricular intervals; SVT: supraventricular tachycardia; VT: ventricular tachycardia.

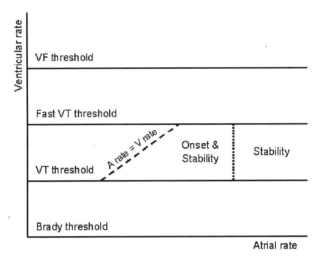

Figure 2.11. Atrial view (algorithm developed by Guidant). It compares atrial with ventricular rate once the threshold for ventricular tachycardia (VT) is reached. Four zones are defined (bradycardia, VT, fast VT, and ventricular fibrillation).

atrioventricular relationship are applied. The association or dissociation of the rhythms is monitored based on the stability criterion. If the ventricular rhythm is stable and the atrial rhythm is unstable, the tachyarrhythmia will be classified as ventricular. If both rhythms are stable, the stability of the atrioventricular relationship is analysed to exclude atrioventricular dissociation. In Guidant dual-chamber devices (Figure 2.11), priority is given to the single-chamber detection criteria onset and stability. An aggressive programming of single-chamber detection criteria in these devices will decrease the sensitivity but increase the specificity of arrhythmia discrimination. The dual-chamber detection criterion 'ventricular rate > atrial rate' can be applied to prevent underdetection of ventricular arrhythmias. The 'Afib threshold' criterion cannot prevent inappropriate arrhythmia classification as priority is given to the stability criterion.

Performance of Dual-chamber Algorithms

The majority of studies conducted with dual-chamber ICDs were restricted to one manufacturer [21–24]. These studies mainly focused on the feasibility and safety of dual-chamber devices, and provided data for improved specificity of arrhythmia detection without compromising the sensitivity for ventricular tachyarrhythmias. The specificity ranged between 66.7 and 93.3% with positive predictive values for ventricular tachyarrhythmias between 87.4 and 98.4%. These data support an actual benefit of dual-chamber devices over single-chamber devices.

Randomized studies comparing single-chamber and dual-chamber ICDs have been performed [25–29]. However, conclusive evidence of the superiority of dual-chamber over single-chamber discrimination has not been proven [30]. The functionality of dual-chamber algorithms is influenced by the accurate determination of the atrial rate [31]. The presence of atrial sensing errors and atrial blanking can result in either misclassification of ventricular arrhythmia as atrial arrhythmia or inappropriate rejection of ventricular arrhythmias.

The Atrioverter: Detection of Atrial Tachyarrhythmias

The philosophy of the atrioverter was different from a conventional ICD [32]. While ICDs had to recognize all ventricular tachyarrhythmias and were prompted to shock when in doubt, the atrioverter was allowed to wait until atrial fibrillation was diagnosed with absolute certainty. A specific device for atrial fibrillation, the Metrix atrioverter system (Incontrol Inc., Redmond, WA, USA), was developed with a two-step detection algorithm. The first algorithm discriminated between a sinus and a non-sinus rhythm, based upon the presence or absence of a 'quiet interval'. The second algorithm, the baseline crossing test (Figure 2.12), was performed on the electrogram obtained between the right atrial electrode and the coronary sinus lead (Figure 2.13).The result of both algorithms was a high sensitivity (100%) for the detection of non-sinus rhythm with a specificity of 96% for atrial fibrillation.

The standalone atrial defibrillator was safe, but required the implantation of a ventricular sensing lead. Mainly under influence of the industry, a dual-chamber device was developed that provided detection and treatment for atrial fibrillation, atrial tachycardia, and ventricular tachyarrhythmias [33].

In the majority of these devices, the detection of atrial arrhythmias is mainly based on rate (with sometimes overlapping zones for atrial tachycardia, flutter, and fibrillation). Evidently, this is not related to real physiology or pathology. For a more accurate classification of atrial tachyarrhythmias, another advanced atrial detection algorithm was developed [34]. This algorithm uses the maximum atrial rate, the standard deviation, and the dispersion of atrial rate to classify unstable and stable atrial arrhythmias.

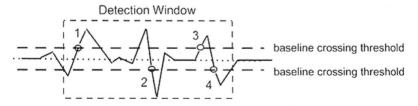

FIGURE 2.12. Atrial fibrillation, as the number of baseline crossings is high.

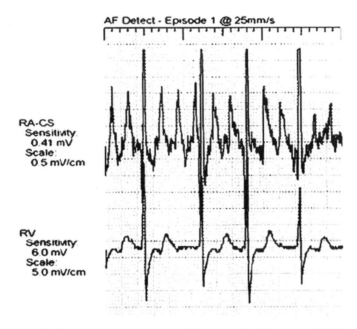

FIGURE 2.13. Atrial fibrillation as detected by the Metrix. Wide band atrial and bipolar near-field right ventricular electrograms.

Morphology-based Algorithms

Some morphology-based algorithms existed in early devices (PDF, Intec and TPM, CPI) as mentioned earlier on. They were never widely used in this era. Medtronic based an algorithm on width of the intracardiac EGM and the slew rate. The ventricular EGM is then classified as narrow or wide by comparing the measured actual width to the programmed value for width threshold value (Figure 2.14). The optimal EGM source for measurements of the EGM width is a far-field configuration between can and coil. The efficacy of the EGM width criterion has been studied by several investigators (Table 2.2). The reported overall sensitivity for detection of ventricular tachycardia was 64.1% [35]. When the data was corrected for stable QRS-complexes in the 12-lead electrocardiogram, the sensitivity was higher on a per-episode basis than on a per-patient basis [35].

The EGM width criterion has several limitations. The criterion cannot be applied in patients with a pre-existing complete bundle branch, which results in underdetection of ventricular tachycardias. Rate-related changes of the electrogram width may result in false-positive detections of ventricular tachycardia. The EGM width is also affected by additional antiarrhythmic drug treatment (class Ic drugs and amiodarone).

Recently, arrhythmia discrimination in the ICD included more advanced morphology algorithms. These algorithms are based on more complex

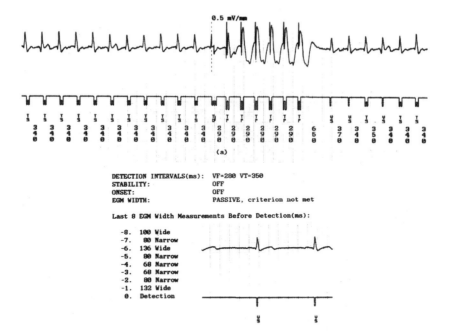

FIGURE 2.14. Ventricular tachycardia with bipolar ventricular electrogram and marker channel. The QRS complexes are similar to the template which is shown in the lower part. Three out of eight complexes preceding the ATP episode are coded as 'Wide'. The criterion was only 'passive' in this case, as detection occurred because of the high rate.

comparisons of electrograms. The 'morphology discrimination' algorithm constructs a quantitative representation of each ventricular complex [36]. This representation is determined by the peak amplitudes, polarities, number of peaks, and the order of peaks. Each ventricular complex during tachycardia is compared to a stored template during the patients' baseline rhythm. The other morphology-based algorithms are the 'vector timing and correlation' algorithm and the 'wavelet transform' algorithm, which are both under clinical investigation [37, 38].

TABLE 2.2. Efficacy of the EGM width criterion.

Investigator	Year	Sensitivity %	Specificity %
Gillberg et al.	1994	100	–
Brachmann et al.	1996	96	76
Duru et al.	1999	–	74
Spehl et al.	1999	100	66
Unterberg et al.	2000	96.7	98.6

References

1. Jordaens L. Recognition of ventricular tachycardia and fibrillation. In Jordaens L, editor. The implantable defibrillator. From concept to clinical reality. Basel: Karger, 1996, pp. 25–33.
2. Brumwell DA, Kroll K, Lehmann MH. The amplifier: sensing the depolarization. In Kroll MW, Lehmann MH, editors. Implantable cardioverter defibrillator therapy: The engineering–clinical interface. London: Kluwer Academic Publishers, 1997, pp. 275–302.
3. Mirowski M, Mower MM, Reid PR. The automatic implantable cardioverter defibrillator. Am Heart J 1980;100:1089–1092.
4. Intec Systems Inc. AID defibrillation summary of initial clinical trials. Third progress report, Pittsburgh, 1982.
5. Kelly PA, Cannom DS, Garan H, Mirabal GS, Harthorne JW, Hurvitz RJ, Vlahakes GJ, Jacobs ML, Ilvento JP, Buckley MJ, et al. The automatic implantable cardioverter-defibrillator: efficacy, complications and survival in patients with malignant ventricular arrhythmias. J Am Coll Cardiol 1988;11:1278–1286.
6. Gabry MD, Brodman R, Johnston D, Frame R, Kim SG, Waspe LE, Fisher JD, Furman S. Automatic implantable cardioverter-defibrillator: patient, survival, battery longevity and shock delivery analysis. J Am Coll Cardiol 1987;9:1349–1356.
7. Winkle RA, Mead RH, Ruder MA, Gaudiani VA, Smith NA, Buch WS, Schmidt P, Shipman T. Long-term outcome with the automatic implantable cardioverter-defibrillator. J Am Coll Cardiol 1989;13:1353–1361.
8. Grimm W, Flores BF, Marchlinski FE. Electrocardiographically documented unnecessary, spontaneous shocks in 241 patients with implantable cardioverter defibrillators. Pacing Clin Electrophysiol 1992;15:1667–1673.
9. Bardy GH, Hofer B, Johnson G, Kudenchuk PJ, Poole JE, Dolack GL, Gleva M, Mitchell R, Kelso D. Implantable transvenous cardioverter-defibrillators. Circulation 1993;87:1152–1168.
10. Theuns DA, Klootwijk APJ, Simoons ML, Jordaens LJ. Clinical variables predicting inappropriate use of implantable cardioverter-defibrillator in patients with coronary artery disease or non-ischemic dilated cardiomyopathy. Am J Cardiol 2005;95:271–274.
11. Swerdlow CD, Chen PS, Kass RM, Allard JR, Peter CT. Discrimination of ventricular tachycardia from sinus tachycardia and atrial fibrillation in a tiered-therapy cardioverter-defibrillator. J Am Coll Cardiol 1994;23:1342–1355.
12. Higgins SL, Lee RS, Kramer RL. Stability: an ICD detection criterion for discriminating atrial fibrillation from ventricular tachycardia. J Cardiovasc Electrophysiol 1995;6:1081–1088.
13. Neuzner J, Pitschner HF, Schlepper M. Programmable VT detection enhancements in implantable cardioverter defibrillator therapy. Pacing Clin Electrophysiol 1995;18:539–547.
14. Kettering K, Dornberger V, Lang R, Vonthein R, Suchalla R, Bosch RF, Mewis C, Eigenberger B, Kuhlkamp V. Enhanced detection criteria in implantable cardioverter defibrillators: sensitivity and specificity of the stability algorithm at different heart rates. Pacing Clin Electrophysiol 2001;24:1325–1333.
15. Nunain SO, Roelke M, Trouton T, Osswald S, Kim YH, Sosa-Suarez G, Brooks DR, McGovern B, Guy M, Torchiana DF, et al. Limitations and late complications of third-generation automatic cardioverter-defibrillators. Circulation 1995;91:2204–2213.

16. Schaumann A, von zur Muhlen F, Gonska BD, Kreuzer H. Enhanced detection criteria in implantable cardioverter-defibrillators to avoid inappropriate therapy. Am J Cardiol 1996;78:42–50.

17. Weber M, Bocker D, Bansch D, Brunn J, Castrucci M, Gradaus R, Breithardt G, Block M. Efficacy and safety of the initial use of stability and onset criteria in implantable cardioverter defibrillators. J Cardiovasc Electrophysiol 1999;10:145–153.

18. Brugada J. Is inappropriate therapy a resolved issue with current implantable cardioverter defibrillators? Am J Cardiol 1999;83:40D–44D.

19. Furman S, Fisher JK, Panizzo F. Necessity of signal processing in tachycardia detection. In: Barold SS, Mugica J, editors. The third decade of cardiac pacing: advances in technology and clinical applications. Mount Kisco, NY: Futura, 1982, pp. 265–274.

20. LeCarpentier GL, Baga JJ, Yang H, Steinman RT, Meissner MD, Lehmann MH. Differentiation of sinus tachycardia from ventricular tachycardia with 1:1 ventriculoatrial conduction in dual chamber implantable cardioverter defibrillators: feasibility of a criterion based on the atrioventricular interval. Pacing Clin Electrophysiol 1994;17:1818–1831.

21. Nair M, Saoudi N, Kroiss D, Letac B. Automatic arrhythmia identification using analysis of the atrioventricular association. Application to a new generation of implantable defibrillators. Circulation 1997;95:967–973.

22. Wilkoff BL, Kuhlkamp V, Volosin K, Ellenbogen K, Waldecker B, Kacet S, Gillberg JM, DeSouza CM. Critical analysis of dual-chamber implantable cardioverter-defibrillator arrhythmia detection: results and technical considerations. Circulation 2001;103:381–386.

23. Theuns D, Klootwijk AP, Kimman GP, Szili-Torok T, Roelandt JR, Jordaens L. Initial clinical experience with a new arrhythmia detection algorithm in dual chamber implantable cardioverter defibrillators. Europace 2001;3:181–186.

24. Kouakam C, Kacet S, Hazard JR, Ferraci A, Mansour H, Defaye P, Davy JM, Lambiez M. Performance of a dual-chamber implantable defibrillator algorithm for discrimination of ventricular from supraventricular tachycardia. Europace 2004;6:32–42.

25. Kuhlkamp V, Dornberger V, Mewis C, Suchalla R, Bosch RF, Seipel L. Clinical experience with the new detection algorithms for atrial fibrillation of a defibrillator with dual chamber sensing and pacing. J Cardiovas Electrophysiol 1999;10:905–915.

26. Deisenhofer I, Kolb C, Nrepepa G, Schreieck J, Karch M, Schmieder S, Zrenner B, Schmitt C. Do current dual chamber cardioverter defibrillators have advantages over conventional single chamber cardioverter defibrillators in reducing inappropriate therapy? A randomized, prospective study. J Cardiovasc Electrophsyiol 2001;12:134–142.

27. Theuns DA, Klootwijk AP, Goedhart DM, Jordaens LJ. Prevention of inappropriate therapy in implantable cardioverter-defibrillators: results of a prospective, randomized study of tachyarrhythmia detection algorithms. J Am Coll Cardiol 2004;44:2362–2367.

28. Bansch D, Steffgen F, Gronefeld G, Wolpert C, Bocker D, Mletzko R, Schoels W, Seidl K, Piel M, Ouyang F, Hohnloser SH, Kuck KH. The 1+1 trial. A prospective trial of a dual- versus a single-chamber implantable defibrillator in patients with slow ventricular tachycardias. Circulation 2004;110:1022–1029.

29. Dorian P, Philippon F, Thibault B, Kimber S, Sterns L, Greene M, Newman D, Gelaznikas R, Barr A. Randomized controlled study of detection enhancements

versus rate-only detection to prevent inappropriate therapy in a dual-chamber implantable cardioverter-defibrillator. Heart Rhythm 2004;1:540–547.

30. Theuns DA, Rivero-Ayerza MJ, Boersma E, Jordaens LJ. Arrhythmia discrimination algorithms to prevent inappropriate therapy: meta-analysis of randomized trials comparing single and dual-chamber ICDs (abstract). Circulation 2005;112 (Suppl II):438.

31. Israel CW, Gronefeld G, Iscolo N, Stoppler C, Hohnloser SH. Discrimination between ventricular and supraventricular tachycardia by dual chamber cardioverter defibrillators: importance of the atrial sensing function. Pacing Clin Electrophysiol 2001;24:183–190.

32. Wellens HJ, Lau CP, Luderitz B, Akhtar M, Waldo AL, Camm AJ, Timmermans C, Tse HF, Jung W, Jordaens L, Ayers G. Atrioverter: an implantable device for the treatment of atrial fibrillation. Circulation 1998;98:1651–1656.

33. Swerdlow CD, Schsls W, Dijkman B, Jung W, Sheth NV, Olson WH, Gunderson BD. Detection of atrial fibrillation and flutter by a dual-chamber implantable cardioverter-defibrillator. For the worldwide Jewel AF investigators. Circulation 2000;101:878–885.

34. Morris MM, KenKnight BH, Lang DJ. Detection of atrial arrhythmia for cardiac rhythm management by implantable devices. J. Electrocardiol 2000;33 Suppl: 133–139.

35. Unterberg C, Stevens J. Vollmann D, Hasenfuss G, Buchwald AB. Long-term clinical experience with the EGM width detection criterion for differentiation of supraventricular and ventricular tachycardia in patients with implantable cardioverter defibrillators. Pacing Clin Electrophysiol 2000;23:1611–1617.

36. Groenefeld GC, Schulte B, Hohnloser SH, Trappe HJ, Korte T, Stellbrink C, Jung W, Meesmann M, Bocker D, Grosse-Meininghaus D, Vogt J, Neuzner J. Morphology discrimination: a beat-to-beat algorithm for the discrimination of ventricular from supraventricular tachycardia by implantable cardioverter defibrillators. Pacing clin Electrophysiol 2001;24:1519–1524.

37. Gold MR, Shorofsky SR, Thompson JA, Kim J, Schwartz M, Bocek J, Lovett EG, Hsu W, Morris MM, Lang DJ. Advanced rhythm discrimination for implantable cardioverter defibrillators using electrogram vector timing and correlation. J Cardiovasc Electrophysiol 2002;13:1092–1097.

38. Swerdlow CD, Brown ML, Lurie K, Zhang J, Wood NM, Olson WH, Gillberg JM. Discrimination of ventricular tachycardia from supraventricular tachycardia by a download wavelet-transform morphology algorithm: a paradigm for development of implantable cardioverter defibrillator detection algorithms. J Cardiovasc Electrophysiol 2002;13:432–441.

3
Device Diagnostics: Interval Tables, Event Counters, Interval Plots, Markers, Electrograms, and New Features

Summary

Diagnostic data of a pulse generator and the patient are now available, offering an array of alphanumerical data. When considering an arrhythmia, data can be clarified with numerical information (intervals), displayed in lists or tables. Event counters can provide information on all kind of events or interventions. Tachograms (or interval plots) display intervals versus time. Electrograms can be taken with different techniques from different channels. Physiological data can be obtained using sensors. All this information can be sent to the patient file, and even become available on the Web for the treating physician.

The ICD contains comprehensive data storage capabilities which offer the physician a possibility to improve patient care. Diagnostic data provide information regarding the function and activity of the pulse generator, which includes information on the battery, the hardware and software, including the lead and the lead-myocardial interface. The ICD has the capability of providing data on arrhythmia occurrence, the cycle length, and date and time of occurrence, with stored electrograms of the events. By examining these data, the physician can determine whether the arrhythmia was a true arrhythmia and whether therapy was appropriate. He can correlate the arrhythmic event with the presence or absence of symptoms and speculate on the electrophysiologic mechanism of the arrhythmia.

Multiple variables may affect the performance of arrhythmia detection by the ICD and one must be familiar with the programmed discrimination algorithms and the various modes of presenting stored diagnostic data. In this chapter, we will discuss the value and limitations of different modes of stored diagnostic information on cardiac arrhythmias.

Interval Tables and Event Counters

The first-generation ICDs provided event counters, displaying device-delivered shocks. The precise diagnosis of the arrhythmia which triggered device therapy and the 'appropriateness' of such therapy was based on the clinical history of the patient, the presence or absence of hemodynamically significant symptoms, or concomitant ECG monitoring. That uncertainty remained present in a large number of events is clear.

The second-generation ICDs stored and showed numerical RR intervals in tables, with or without device activity markers. This stored information allowed analysis of the rate of the arrhythmia preceding and following ICD therapy. Differentiation of arrhythmias was based on the regularity of RR intervals. Irregular intervals suggested atrial fibrillation, while regular intervals could indicate sinus tachycardia, atrial flutter, or atrial tachycardia as well as ventricular tachycardia. As was known from clinical observations, even monomorphic ventricular tachycardia may demonstrate irregular intervals at its onset, which makes it difficult to differentiate it from atrial fibrillation with this kind of information. Further, the detected intervals may include appropriately detected intervals or inappropriately detected or oversensed events due to intracardiac or extracardiac signals. As a consequence, arrhythmia diagnosis based on RR intervals alone remains associated with uncertainty[1].

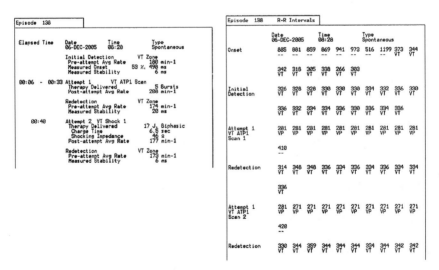

FIGURE 3.1. Example of an episode text and the corresponding interval table displaying the RR intervals preceding and following device therapy for ventricular tachycardia (VT). After the first attempt of antitachycardia pacing (ATP), the device redetected RR intervals in the tachycardia detection zone. These RR intervals confirmed redetection of VT and triggered the next attempt with ATP to terminate VT. The episode text does not give details of the delivered attempts of ATP.

```
BIOTRONIK    SWM  1000
   Rel I-GAV.O.U/1          20.05.1999 10:39

        System Status

   Num Capacitor Reforms:        1
   Last Capacitor Reform.:       09.11.98

                                 Cleared:
                                 01.04.99
   ATP Therapies                 2              4
   VF Shocks                     0              5
   VT Shocks                     0              0
   Aborted VF Shocks             0              0
   Aborted VT Shocks             0              0
   Manual Shocks                 0              0
   Discrimination Successes      0              1
   Mode Conversions              0              0
   % Atrial Paced                66             23
   % Ventricular Paced           1              55

   Battery Status                BOL
```

FIGURE 3.2. Example of event counters. The first column displays device performance since the last interrogation. The last column displays the total performance since implantation.

In current devices, interval tables are still available. They can provide additional information to assess the outcome of delivered antitachycardia pacing or shock therapies (Figure 3.1).

ICD diagnostics include information on the battery status, energy consumption, lead impedance, and the integrity of the high-voltage shock circuit. Event counters can help to assess the overall performance of the device. The counters provide information on pacemaker function such as the percentage of paced and sensed events. For tachyarrhythmias, the event counters provide the number of delivered therapies, and aborted or inhibited therapies (Figures 3.2 and 3.3).

Electrograms

With third-generation devices, the most significant advance in diagnostic information was the storage of intracardiac electrogram recordings. This diagnostic information included recording of RR intervals preceding and following device therapy, and stored electrograms with real-time markers of arrhythmias triggering device therapy. The current generation of devices can be programmed to record events from different electrogram sources. The electrograms can be recorded from the pair of electrodes used for rate sensing (near-field), the defibrillation coils (far-field or wide-band), or both. Both

Arrhythmia / Therapy statistics

Last treated episode: VT 07/Feb/2006 10:22

Total number of shocks since beginning of life (without EPS) : 5

ARRHYTHMIAS	FV / Fast VT	VT	Slow VT	Others
Detection	2	6	0	0
Termination by ATP	0 (0%)	3 (50%)	0	0
Termination by Shock	2 (100%)	3 (50%)	0	0
Spontaneous arrest	0 (0%)	0 (0%)	0	0
THERAPIES	**FV / Fast VT**	**VT**	**Slow VT**	**Others**
Delivered(%effective)	2	9	0	0
ATP	0	6 (50%)	0	0
Shock	2 (100%)	3 (100%)	0	0
34J shock	0	0	0	0

Unsuccessful ATP on Fast VT   : 0

Pacing / Sensing Statistic

PMT : 0   **Time in MS** : 09h 09min   **ModeSwitch** : 6

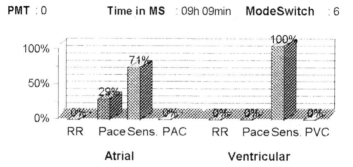

FIGURE 3.3. Example of event counters with separate statistics for arrhythmia therapy and pacemaker performance.

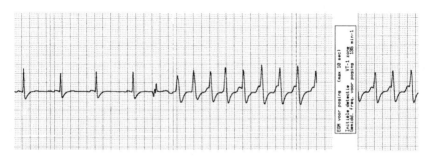

FIGURE 3.4. Stored bipolar far-field ventricular electrogram demonstrating a change in electrogram morphology during ventricular tachycardia as compared to the supraventricular baseline rhythm. The atrial activity is reflected on the far-field ventricular electrogram.

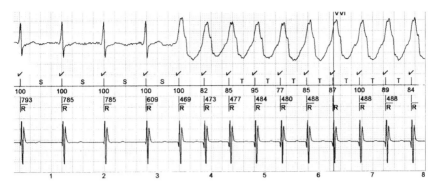

FIGURE 3.5. Real-time registration in a single-chamber device. From top to bottom, surface electrocardiogram lead II, device activity channel with marker annotations, and near-field ventricular electrogram. Note the subtle change in the near-field ventricular electrogram morphology: the first negative peak is more pronounced during VT compared to sinus rhythm.

electrogram sources have advantages and disadvantages. Near-field ventricular electrograms show no atrial activity, which could result in an inability to diagnose the arrhythmia triggering the device. However, they can provide information on detection problems such as the presence of over- or under-sensing of signals. In contrast, far-field electrograms have the advantage that they resemble the conventional surface electrocardiogram. The far-field electrogram can reflect atrial activity and ventricular electrogram morphology changes, which both can be helpful for arrhythmia diagnosis by the physician (Figure 3.4).

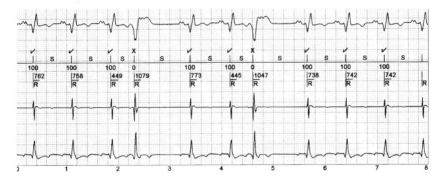

FIGURE 3.6. Real-time registration in a single-chamber device. From top to bottom, surface electrocardiogram lead II, device activity channel with marker annotations, near-field ventricular electrogram, and far-field ventricular electrogram. The atrial activity is reflected on the far-field ventricular electrogram. Two ventricular premature beats, the 4th and 6th beat, show a subtle change in the far-field electrogram. The amplitude of the electrogram is increased as compared to the baseline ventricular electrogram during sinus rhythm. The morphology of the ventricular premature beat has a "QRS" pattern in the near-field ventricular electrogram, while the ventricular electrogram morphology has a "Rs" pattern during sinus rhythm.

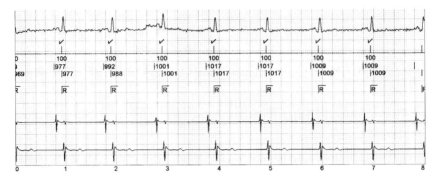

FIGURE 3.7. Real-time registration in a dual-chamber device. From top to bottom, surface electrocardiogram lead II, device activity channel with marker annotations, atrial electrogram, and near-field ventricular electrogram. The real-time registration shows sinus rhythm.

The correlation of electrograms with markers, rate characteristics, and RR-interval stability improves the understanding of electrograms to diagnose the arrhythmia triggering the device. The presence of device activity markers allows the physician to analyze how the device interacts with arrhythmias.

Electrograms can be displayed online (in real time) on the programmer (with a printer) or can be recorded on a conventional ECG recorder. Some examples of online electrograms are shown in Figures 3.5–3.8.

If electrograms are stored in the ICD, they can improve the retrospective analysis of events. To save energy, only a limited number of episodes are completely shown, and sometimes only short strips ("snapshots") can be obtained. Today, it is possible to retrieve the electrogram remotely from the patient, via a GSM, or the Internet. This form of telemedicine will certainly change our attitude and possibilities for follow-up (Figure 3.9).

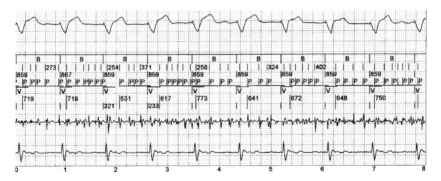

FIGURE 3.8. Real-time registration in a dual-chamber device. From top to bottom, surface electrocardiogram lead II, device activity channel with marker annotations, atrial electrogram, and near-field ventricular electrogram. The atrial electrogram shows multiple events. The real-time registration shows atrial fibrillation and ventricular pacing.

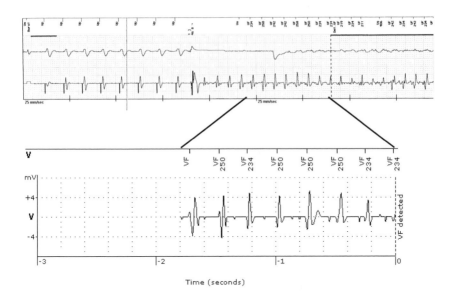

FIGURE 3.9. Example of a transtelephonically transmitted stored ventricular electrogram with the accompanying electrogram, which was obtained at interrogation of the device (surface and far-field). The transmitted electrogram shows a snapshot of ventricular fibrillation during intra-operative testing of defibrillation efficacy. The transmitted electrogram resembles the stored far-field electrogram as obtained during intra-operative testing.

Interval Plots (Tachograms)

The interval plot is a graphical presentation of the detected intervals (ms) plotted versus time (sec). The detected intervals preceding arrhythmia detection, during the arrhythmia, and after delivered ICD therapy are displayed. The plot shows V-V and A-A intervals with different symbols (e.g. closed circles "●" or open squares "□"). In the interval plot, the

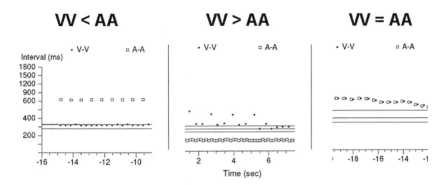

FIGURE 3.10. Application of rate branches in relation to interval plots (Medtronic devices). With VV and AA, intervals are shown, not rate.

programmed rate cutoffs for the detection zones are displayed as horizontal lines and their values are printed at the top of the interval plot. The time "0" seconds represents the fulfilled tachycardia detection.

By analyzing the relationship of atrial and ventricular activities, the interpretation of the interval plot can provide a fast diagnosis of the arrhythmia triggering device therapy, especially in dual-chamber defibrillators. Based on the comparison of atrial and ventricular intervals, tachyarrhythmias can be roughly divided into three rate branches: ventricular rate > atrial rate (VV < AA), ventricular rate < atrial rate (VV > AA), and ventricular rate = atrial rate (VV = AA). Figure 3.10 shows the application of the different branches in relation to interval plots. The majority of ventricular tachyarrhythmias have ventricular rates faster than the atrial rate (branch VV < AA). This dissociated atrioventricular conduction is characterized by two separate tracks of the atrial and ventricular rate/interval.

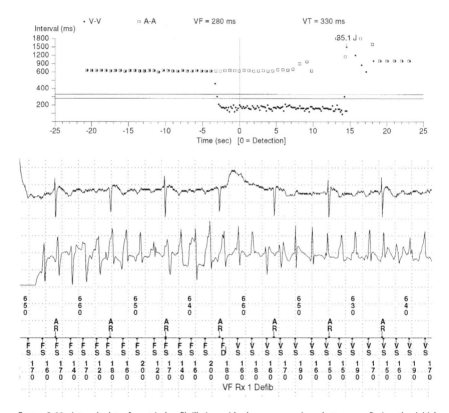

FIGURE 3.11. Interval plot of ventricular fibrillation with the accompanying electrogram. During the initial rhythm, the interval plot shows that each ventricular activity is preceded by an atrial activity. The ventricular intervals have a cycle length of ≈ 600 ms. At the onset of the tachyarrhythmia, there is a sudden decrease of ventricular intervals, while the atrial intervals remain constant. The ventricular intervals have a mean cycle length of ≈ 170 ms, the atrial intervals of ≈ 600 ms.

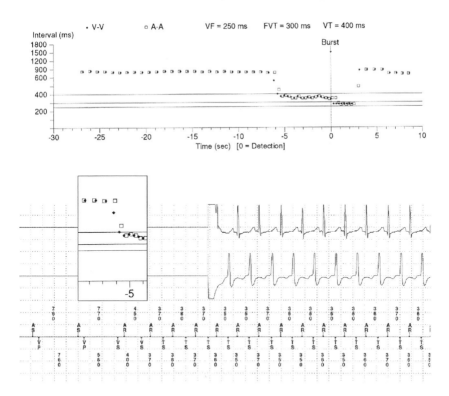

FIGURE 3.12. Interval plot of ventricular tachycardia with 1:1 retrograde atrioventricular conduction, and the accompanying electrogram. During the initial rhythm, the interval plot shows that each ventricular activity is preceded by an atrial activity. The ventricular intervals have a cycle length of ≈ 700 ms. At the onset of tachyarrhythmia, there is a sudden decrease of the ventricular intervals followed by a decrease in atrial intervals. During the tachyarrhythmia, each ventricular activity is followed by an atrial activity. The ventricular intervals have a mean cycle length of ≈ 360 ms.

Some examples of interval plots of arrhythmias recorded in dual-chamber devices are shown in Figures 3.11–3.16.

Event Markers, Marker Channels™, Status Channel

With third-generation devices, it became possible to display real-time data and stored data using several tabular or graphical options. One interesting, simple, and easy-to-use option is to show timing events (for pacing, sensing of normal beats, sensing of arrhythmias – tachycardia, fast tachycardia, fibrillation-, the starting of capacitor charging, the delivery of therapy -ATP or shocks-). These events can be displayed as single, double, or multiple lines above and/or below a baseline, with different calibrations according to the event. Figure 3.17 shows the different calibrations for ELA-Medical defibrillators.

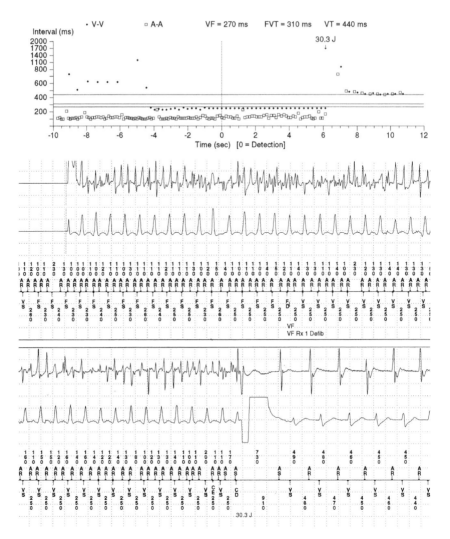

FIGURE 3.13. Interval plot of ventricular tachycardia during atrial fibrillation, and the accompanying electrogram. The initial rhythm is sensed atrial, ventricular paced with a cycle length of $\approx 600\,\text{ms}$. At the onset of the tachyarrhythmia, there is a sudden decrease of ventricular cycle length ($\approx 260\,\text{ms}$), and the ventricular intervals are stable during the tachyarrhythmia. The delivered shock terminates the ventricular tachycardia, and restores sinus rhythm as well.

In the majority of current devices, the device activity is annotated by markers (Table 3.1). The markers represent the ICD's classification for each detected event by letter symbols.

TABLE 3.1. Most important marker annotations for normal rhythm and for tachyarrhythmias. Device activity markers are summarised for Biotronik, Guidant, Medtronic, and St Jude Medical ICDs.

	Manufacturer			
	Biotronik	Guidant	Medtronic	St Jude Medical
Atrial pace	AP	AP	AP	A
Atrial refractory sense	AR	(AS)	AR	A
Atrial sense	AS	AS	AS	P
Ventricular pace	VP	VP	VP	V
Ventricular sense	VS	VS	VS	R
Ventricular fibrillation	F	VF	VF	F
Ventricular tachycardia	VT	VT	TS	T
Ventricular tachycardia		VT-1, VT	TS, TF	T, TB

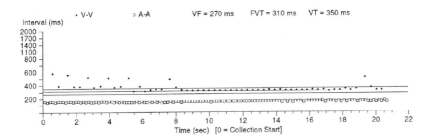

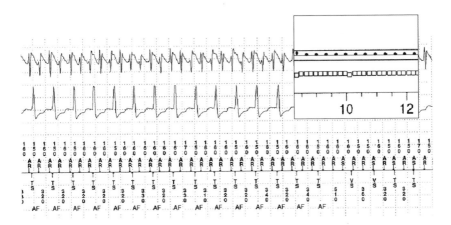

FIGURE 3.14. Interval plot of atrial flutter, and the accompanying electrogram. The interval plot shows stable atrial intervals with a cycle length of ≈ 160 ms. In the interval plot, at time "8 seconds", the ventricular rhythm becomes stable. During this stable rhythm, each ventricular interval has two atrial activities as shown in the snapshot.

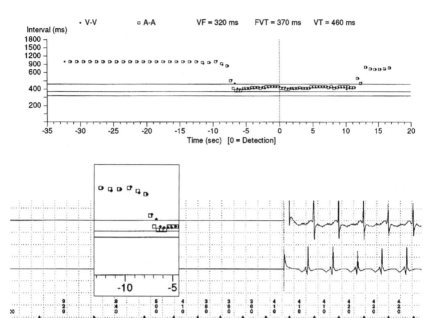

FIGURE 3.15. Interval plot of atrial tachycardia, and the accompanying electrogram. During the initial rhythm, the interval plot shows that each ventricular activity is preceded by an atrial activity. The ventricular intervals have a cycle length of ≈ 950 ms. At the onset of tachyarrhythmia, there is a sudden decrease of the atrial intervals followed by a decrease in ventricular intervals (see snapshot). During the onset of the tachyarrhythmia, the atrioventricular conduction is increased until the arrhythmia reaches a stable cycle length of ≈ 420 ms. During the tachyarrhythmia, each ventricular activity is preceded by an atrial activity.

New Features

Physiologic Data

The increased storage capability of cardiac resynchronization therapy (CRT) devices allow beat-to-beat analysis that enables continuous sampling of physiologic parameters. Device-based monitoring of heart rate and time-domain parameters of heart rate variability (HRV) can be helpful in evaluating the therapeutic effects of CRT in heart failure patients. Diminished HRV and an increased mean heart rate in patients with heart failure are associated with a poor prognosis [2].

Continuous monitoring of the thoracic impedance is used since a long time to increase pacing rate; it became available again in some devices to assess fluid overload (Figure 3.18). Detection of decreased thoracic impedance could lead to early diagnosis of volume overload [3].

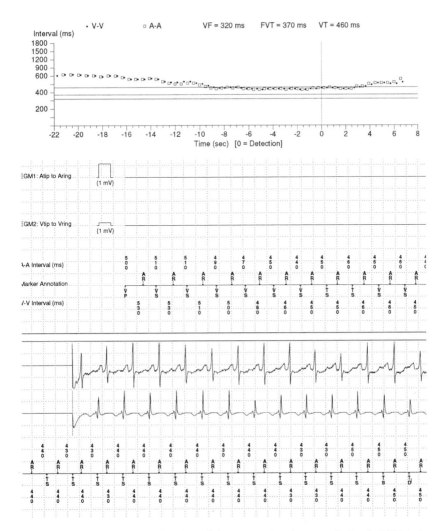

Figure 3.16. Interval plot of sinus tachycardia, and the accompanying electrogram. During the initial rhythm, the interval plot shows that each ventricular activity is preceded by an atrial activity. The ventricular intervals have a cycle length of ≈ 450 ms. The interval plot shows a gradual increase in ventricular rate. During the tachyarrhythmia, the atrioventricular conduction gradually increases until the arrhythmia reaches a stable cycle length of ≈ 440–450 ms. During the tachyarrhythmia, each ventricular activity is preceded by an atrial activity.

Telemetered Data

As the society is moving towards a much more ambulatory approach of patient care, the idea of remote monitoring is very attractive. When applied to ICD therapy, supervision of both clinical and technical aspects becomes possible [4, 5]. Table 3.2 gives an indication of the possibilities. Diagnostic data such as the numbers of aborted and delivered ICD therapies are an indicator

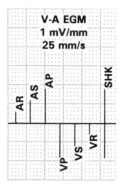

FIGURE 3.17. Marker calibrations in ELA Medical defibrillators.

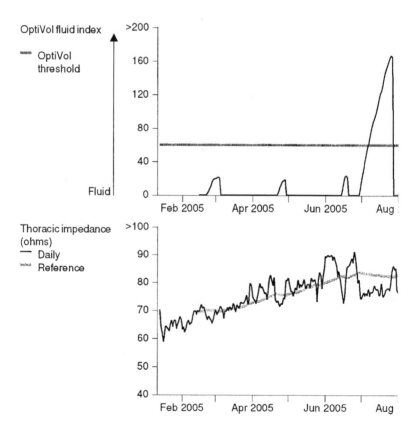

FIGURE 3.18. Example of monitored diagnostic data in a cardiac resynchronization device. In July 2005, a decrease in thoracic impedance is paralleled by an increase in the fluid index (Medtronic).

TABLE 3.2. Stored clinical and technical information in the device, with a potential for remote monitoring.

Possibilities of diagnostic and therapeutic information with Home Monitoring with actual arrhythmia devices	
Clinical Information	*General*
	– Electrogram in actual rhythm
	– Heart rate
	– Heart rate variability
	Pacing related
	– Percentage atrial pacing
	– Percentage AV synchrony
	– Percentage ventricular pacing
	– Number of mode switches
	Tachyarrhythmia related
	– Number of AT episodes
	– Number of AF episodes
	– Number of VT episodes
	– Number of VF episodes
	– Number of nonsustained episodes
	– Number of delivered ICD therapies
	– Number of aborted ICD therapies
	– Electrogram of arrhythmia
	Sensor related
	– Motion
	– Respiration
	– Impedance
	– Pressure
Technical Information	Battery status and voltage
	Shock impedance
	P- and R-wave amplitudes
	Autocapture thresholds
	Impedance of pace/sense leads

of the total incidence of tachyarrhythmias. Frequently recurring episodes of ventricular tachyarrhythmias in patients may indicate increasing instability and progression of cardiac disease.

Conclusion

In Chapter 6 we will present a series of examples of electrograms which were obtained with a variety of devices. In some cases, ancillary diagnostic data provided the information for the definite arrhythmia diagnosis. The more information that was present, the less necessary additional surface ECGs became.

References

1. Marchlinski FE, Buxton AE, Flores BF. The automatic implantable cardioverter defibrillator: Followup and complications. In: El-Sherif N, Samet P, editors. Cardiac pacing and electrophysiology. Orlando, Fl: Grune and Stratton, 1990, pp. 743–758.
2. Fantoni C, Raffa S, Regoli F, et al. Cardiac resynchronization therapy improves heart rate profile and heart rate variability of patients with moderate to severe heart failure. J Am Coll Cardiol 2005;46:1875–1882.
3. Yu CM, Wang L, Chau E, et al. Intrathoracic impedance monitoring in patients with heart failure: correlation with fluid status and feasibility of early warning preceding hospitalization. Circulation 2005;112:841–848.
4. Theuns DA, Res JC, Jordaens LJ. Home monitoring in ICD therapy: future perspectives. Europace 2003;5:139–142.
5. Schoenfeld MH, Reynolds DW. Sophisticated remote implantable cardioverter-defibrillator follow-up: a status report. Pacing Clin Electrophysiol 2005;28:235–240.

4
Understanding Stored Electrograms

Summary
Stored electrograms in ICDs have not only improved patient management, but also increased our understanding of tachyarrhythmias. Stored electrograms are usually analyzed visually by physicians. This analysis can also be performed in a methodological way by using building blocks with physiologic information. Each block contains specific timing- or morphology-based characteristics of arrhythmias. A systematic approach is proposed, which can help physicians and technicians to avoid a biased analysis.

This chapter will provide an approach for the analysis of stored electrograms. It has been proven that experienced physicians still interpret electrograms more accurately than the device itself [1, 2]. However, this requires a thorough knowledge of the standard interpretation of ECGs and underlying arrhythmia mechanisms. Some fundamental basics remain the same, whether the ECG is derived from the surface or from intracardiac electrodes. When good electrograms are available, device diagnostics should be superior to the 12-lead ECG (Figure 4.1).

Information is not always complete (e.g. when no atrial lead is present), and the physician then has to make assumptions to narrow down the differential diagnosis. To help in this process, we propose the application of blocks with physiologic information to interpret stored electrograms.

Electrogram Sources

The current generation of devices can be programmed to record events from different electrogram sources. The electrograms can be recorded from the pair of electrodes used for rate sensing (near-field), the defibrillation coils (far-field or wide-band), or both (Figure 4.2). The pulse generator can be used as part of the shock circuit, and become an electrode to generate the electrogram as well.

Each type of electrogram has advantages and disadvantages. Near-field ventricular electrograms ("rate") show no atrial activity, which limits the ability to discriminate between atrial and ventricular tachyarrhythmias. However, they can provide information on detection problems such as the

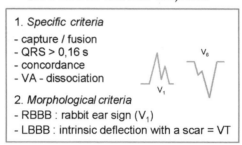

ECG criteria for ventricular tachycardia

1. *Specific criteria*
- capture / fusion
- QRS > 0,16 s
- concordance
- VA - dissociation

2. *Morphological criteria*
- RBBB : rabbit ear sign (V₁)
- LBBB : intrinsic deflection with a scar = VT

FIGURE 4.1. Conventional criteria for differentiating VT from SVT with aberration during wide QRS tachycardia (modified from reference 18). It becomes clear that these criteria will not always be applicable to device electrograms, as they lack for instance some of the morphology data available on the surface. The presence, absence, or timing of atrial activity will be far more accurate when an intracardiac atrial signal is available.

presence of over- or undersensing of different signals. In contrast, far-field ventricular electrograms ("shock") have the advantage of showing atrial activity and reflecting changes in electrogram morphology as well. Both types (rate and shock) can be helpful in arrhythmia diagnosis by the physician. Far-field ventricular electrograms resemble the surface ECG, with all associated advantages and uncertainty. Importantly, the electrogram features should be programmed to have a maximal benefit for visual analysis. Far-field ventricular electrograms are generally preferable. Electrograms should be stored in such a way that the arrhythmia onset is kept in the memory.

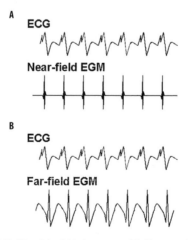

FIGURE 4.2. Examples of near-field (A) and far-field electrograms (B). The terms "rate" and "shock" electrogram are commonly used to describe each respective type.

Visual Analysis of Stored Electrograms

In general, tachyarrhythmia detection algorithms use combinations of information derived from atrial and ventricular data. This applies for tachycardia differentiation in general electrocardiography, but is improved for antitachycardia devices which have more precise diagnostic information from intracardiac signals. Tachyarrhythmia discrimination in devices is performed in a stepwise process using sets or "blocks" of physiologically relevant information. Each set describes a specific timing or morphological aspect which contains characteristics of tachyarrhythmias. This results in a device diagnosis which is not always accurate, but is aimed at detecting all ventricular tachyarrythmias, and therefore accepts to a certain level inappropriate therapies for supraventricular rhythms. These blocks with physiological information can also be applied in visual analysis of stored electrograms, derived from intracardiac or thoracic leads and devices. This approach can be considered as a tool to improve the device diagnostics.

Single Chamber Devices

In single chamber devices, information "blocks" are derived from the sensed ventricular activity (Table 4.1). Each block contains information about the tachyarrhythmia, but it is evident that limitations are inherent to single chamber devices, certainly for discrimination between atrial and ventricular tachyarrhythmias.

VV Intervals (or Ventricular Rate)

Ventricular rate (the inverse of VV interval or ventricular cycle length) is a very sensitive parameter to detect all ventricular tachyarrhythmias. However it has a low specificity as it overlaps with all other tachycardias (sinus, atrial, and supraventricular). Nevertheless, rate-only detection was associated with a better outcome than detection based on early morphology criteria [3]. Rate zones are now increasingly used, and divided into slow, normal, fast (or VT), very fast VT, and ventricular fibrillation. Evidently, this is not based on electrophysiology, but just on arbitrary definitions.

TABLE 4.1. Available information blocks in single chamber devices.

- VV intervals (or ventricular rate)
- electrogram width
- electrogram morphology
- VV interval stability
- sudden onset

Electrogram Width

Far-field ventricular electrograms are used to measure the electrogram width. This interesting feature, with a link to the 12-lead criteria, has limitations, as the electrogram width should be compared to width during normal baseline or sinus rhythm. This criterion is not applicable in patients with complete bundle branch block [4]. Another shortcoming of this criterion is the change in electrogram width due to additional antiarrhythmic drug therapy [5]. In devices this criterion is linked to slew rate, which might indeed give a clue to the diagnosis of VT, as it is assumed that a long intrinsic deflection is associated with structural heart disease [6].

Electrogram Morphology

The widely used block "ventricular electrogram morphology", which is related to QRS width, or includes QRS width, is mainly based on the premise that the electrogram morphology will change during ventricular tachyarrhythmias as compared to a supraventricular baseline rhythm (Figure 4.3).

A distinct change in the electrogram morphology was identified in 93% of induced ventricular tachycardias [7]. The analysis of far-field electrograms permits a more accurate arrhythmia classification. However, the development of rate-dependent aberrancy during supraventricular tachycardia alters the electrogram morphology as compared to baseline sinus rhythm [8]. Specifically, a change in electrogram morphology was predominantly observed at recording sites ipsilateral to the bundle branch block [9].

Stability

The information block "VV interval stability" is used to discriminate between monomorphic ventricular tachycardia, characterized by regular ventricular intervals, and atrial fibrillation, characterized by irregular ventricular intervals [10]. The limitation of this block is the regular ventricular response during atrial tachyarrhythmias with fixed N:1 atrioventricular conduction, as supraventricular and atrial tachycardia, and typically, 2:1 atrial flutter. Another limitation is the increased stability of VV intervals during atrial fibrillation with very fast ventricular response [11].

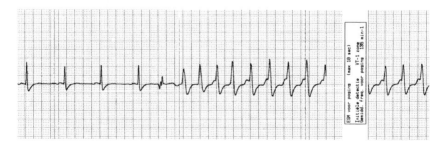

FIGURE 4.3. Stored bipolar shock electrogram demonstrating a change in electrogram morphology during ventricular tachycardia as compared to the supraventricular baseline rhythm. (Guidant, model Mini IV)

Sudden Onset

The block "sudden onset" can be used to discriminate sudden onset ventricular tachyarrhythmias from sinus tachycardia which is characterized by a gradual onset. However, sudden onset may not be specific for ventricular tachyarrhythmias as atrial or supraventricular tachycardia can be initiated by a premature beat and show a sudden onset pattern. This feature has been studied extensively [10, 12, 13].

Combined Criteria

Appropriate interpretation of stored electrograms in single chamber devices is not only based on changes in one information block. The information of the electrogram morphology is combined with information on the rate of the arrhythmia, the onset, and the stability of the arrhythmia. The recording of device activity markers (marker channel) provides additional information and requires little memory capacity (Figure 4.4).

It has been demonstrated that the combined use of electrogram morphology, rate characteristics, and VV interval stability allowed a correct diagnosis to be made in 97% of the events [14]. A flow chart displaying a way of analyzing arrhythmias is shown in Figure 4.5. It also suggests that limitations remain present even with the combined information.

Dual Chamber Devices

The visual analysis of stored electrograms from dual chamber devices applies information blocks based on atrial and ventricular physiological data (Table 4.2). Blocks derived from the ventricular activity are similar to those used in single chamber devices. Information blocks with clinical data of atrial activity are "AA stability", "atrial cycle length" and "atrial electrogram

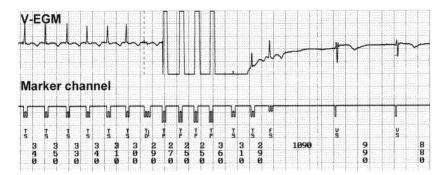

FIGURE 4.4. Stored bipolar electrogram showing ventricular tachycardia (VT) with regular ventricular intervals detected in the programmed tachycardia detection zone. The programmed tachycardia detection (TD) is fulfilled and subsequently antitachycardia pacing (ATP) is delivered. The ventricular electrogram morphology is significantly different during tachycardia as compared to the restored baseline rhythm. Markers: FS = fibrillation sensing; Rx = therapy; TD = tachycardia detected; TP = tachycardia pacing; TS = tachycardia sensing; VS = ventricular sensing sensing; VT = ventricular tachycardia. (Medtronic Jewel, model 7219)

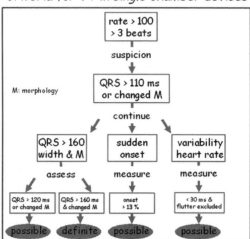

FIGURE 4.5. Criteria that can be used for visual interpretation of stored electrograms in a single-chamber device. When criteria are combined, better results can be expected.

morphology". These blocks can be used to identify the presence and the character of atrial tachyarrhythmias.

AA Intervals (or Atrial Rate)

Atrial rate (the inverse of AA interval or atrial cycle length) has been used in different ways to define atrial tachyarrhythmias in devices [3]. Rate zones to classify atrial and supraventricular arrhythmias face similar limitations as rate zones at the ventricular level. In particular, the overlap between sinus and supraventricular tachycardia and between atrial tachycardia and atrial flutter is unclear [15, 16].

TABLE 4.2. Available information blocks in dual chamber devices.

- VV intervals (or ventricular rate)
- VV interval stability
- AA intervals (or atrial rate)
- AA interval stability
- V electrogram width
- V electrogram morphology
- A electrogram width
- A electrogram morphology
- AV conduction pattern
- AV dissociation
- sudden onset
- chamber of origin

AA Stability

Flutter is strictly regular. This also applies for supraventricular tachycardia. Standard deviation has been used in algorithms to better define atrial fibrillation, where standard deviation (of atrial activity) is high [17].

Atrial Electrogram Width/Morphology

Activation of the atrium, different from the normal activation, is present in all supraventricular arrhythmias, except in sinus tachycardia and ectopic or re-entrant tachycardia arising near the sinus node. In (AV-) nodal tachycardia, the retrograde P-wave can be less wide than in other situations, as the activation of the atria is initiated from the inter-atrial septum, without the normal interatrial conduction delay. The same is observed in the presence of a septal bypass tract or when VA conduction occurs during ventricular tachycardia.

AV Dissociation

The absence of a relation between atrial and ventricular electrogram has always been a cornerstone in arrhythmia analysis ('cherchez le P'). This becomes very easy with intracardiac atrial electrograms. Analysis of the atrioventricular (AV) relationship can easily be performed when information from both levels is available. A far-field signal which might (or might not) display atrial activity can lead to the same pitfalls as the frequent misinterpretation of the 12-lead ECG.

AV Conduction Pattern

Wenckebach patterns, fixed 2:1 block, and complete block in both directions can be described. In flutter some complex patterns can be observed.

'AV conduction pattern' can be used to discriminate between atrial and ventricular tachyarrhythmias. The majority of atrial tachyarrhythmias have a consistent AV conduction pattern, which can be different from sinus rhythm. Ventricular tachyarrhythmias with stable retrograde 1:1 ventriculoatrial (VA) conduction are not uncommon [18].

Chamber of Origin

Another helpful block is the "chamber of origin", which can be used to discriminate between atrial and ventricular tachyarrhythmias with 1:1 AV or VA conduction by identification of atrial activity preceding ventricular activity or vice versa.

All information blocks with relevant data can serve as a tool for analysis of stored electrograms. The use of specific physiologic blocks and the order or combination is illustrated in Figure 4.6, and will most often lead to a comparison of the atrial and ventricular rates.

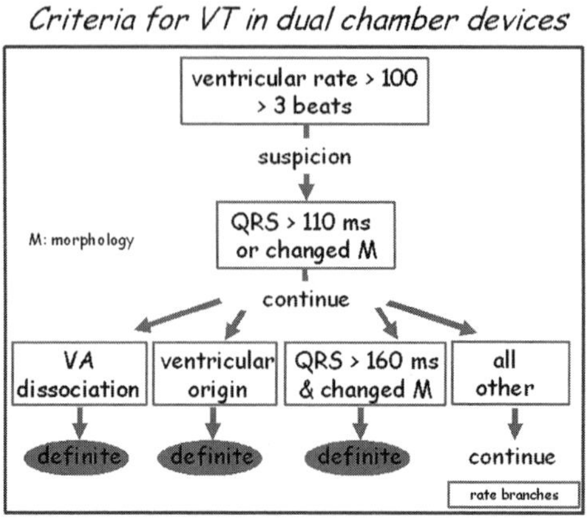

Criteria for VT in dual chamber devices

FIGURE 4.6. Criteria that can be used for visual interpretation of stored electrograms in a dual-chamber device. It is easy to understand that a definite diagnosis is more readily reached than in the situation in Figure 4.5. When no definite diagnosis is reached it is suggested to proceed to the rate classification based upon the atrial and ventricular rates.

Application of Information Blocks in Relation to Rate Branches

Based on the comparison of atrial and ventricular rate, tachyarrhythmias can be roughly divided into three rate branches: ventricular rate > atrial rate, ventricular rate < atrial rate, and ventricular rate = atrial rate (Figure 4.7). Unfortunately, the abbreviations VV and AA as used by manufacturers usually stands for intervals (cycle length) and not for rate (which is misleading when we talk about rate branches).

Ventricular Rate > Atrial Rate

In the majority of ventricular tachyarrhythmias, the ventricular rate is faster than the atrial rate (Figure 4.8). In this rate branch, the timing-based physiologic blocks "atrial rate", "ventricular rate", "AV dissociation" and "VV interval stability" are applicable. The block "ventricular electrogram morphology" can be used to discriminate between monomorphic and polymorphic ventricular tachycardias. Monomorphic ventricular tachycardia has a constant cycle length, beat-to-beat variation < 10%, and a uniform electrogram morphology during the tachycardia [19].

Ventricular Rate < Atrial Rate

Compared to the former group, the rate branch "ventricular rate < atrial rate" is more complex. Atrial tachyarrhythmias within this rate branch can be atrial fibrillation, atrial flutter, or atrial tachycardia with stable N:1 AV conduction. The occurrence of ventricular tachyarrhythmias in this rate branch is also

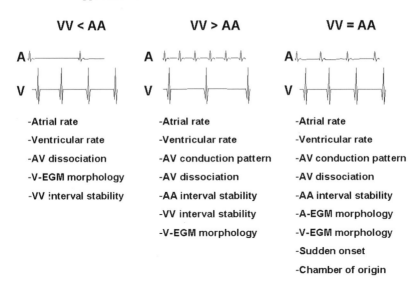

FIGURE 4.7. Available information blocks with relevant data in dual chamber devices; application in relation to the relative rate of atria and ventricles. VV and AA stand for the cycle length or interval, not for rate.

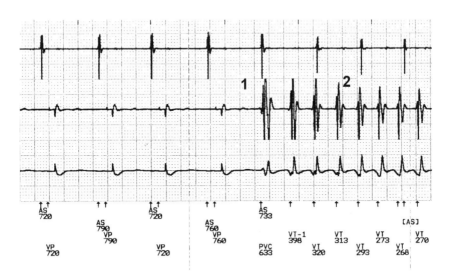

FIGURE 4.8. Stored bipolar electrograms showing ventricular tachycardia (VT). Rhythm strip from top to bottom: atrial, ventricular, and shock electrogram. A ventricular premature beat (1) initiates VT (2) with regular ventricular intervals detected in the programmed tachycardia detection zone. During VT, the ventricular rate is faster than the atrial rate. Markers: AS = atrial sensing; PVC = premature ventricular complex; VP = ventricular pacing; VT = ventricular tachycardia window. (Guidant Prizm DR, model 1861)

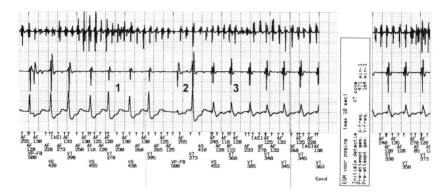

FIGURE 4.9. Stored bipolar electrograms demonstrating double tachycardia, which is ventricular tachycardia (VT) during atrial fibrillation (AF). Rhythm strip from top to bottom: atrial, ventricular, and shock electrogram. The atrial electrogram shows atrial fibrillation. A ventricular premature beat (2) initiates VT (3). During VT, the morphology of the ventricular and shock electrograms change as compared to baseline rhythm (1). Markers: AF = atrial fibrillation window; AS = atrial sensing; VP-FB = ventricular pacing, fallback; VS = ventricular sensing; VT = ventricular tachycardia window. (Guidant, Renewal II, model H155)

known as "double tachycardia", most often atrial fibrillation and ventricular tachycardia. On the atrial level, the blocks "atrial rate", "AA interval stability", and "AV conduction pattern" can be used to identify the type of atrial tachyarrhythmia. A regular atrial rhythm is usually found during atrial flutter or tachycardia.

For the identification of ventricular tachycardia, combinations of blocks "AV dissociation", "VV interval stability", and "ventricular electrogram morphology" are used (Figure 4.9). The ventricular electrogram morphology and stability of ventricular intervals are applicable for identification of ventricular tachycardia during atrial fibrillation. The blocks "AV dissociation" and "ventricular electrogram morphology" are suitable for identification of ventricular tachycardia during atrial flutter or tachycardia. Atrial flutter or tachycardia with stable N:1 AV conduction have a consistent AV conduction pattern. This AV conduction pattern will change when ventricular tachycardia is present (Figure 4.10). The physiologic block "VV interval stability" is not applicable during atrial tachyarrhythmias with stable N:1 AV conduction as the ventricular response is regular.

Ventricular Rate = Atrial Rate

The rate branch "ventricular rate = atrial rate" consists of tachyarrhythmias with 1:1 AV or VA conduction. In this rate branch, the AV conduction relationship plays an important role. The atrial tachyarrhythmias (i.e. sinus and atrial tachycardia) have a consistent AV conduction pattern. On the other hand, ventricular tachyarrhythmias with stable retrograde 1:1 VA conduction also have a consistent VA conduction pattern. To discriminate between atrial

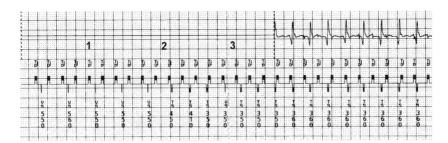

Figure 4.10. Detection of double tachycardia, which is ventricular tachycardia (VT) during atrial flutter (AFl). The marker channel demonstrates appropriately detected AFl (1) with a consistent atrioventricular (AV) conduction pattern. A ventricular premature beat (2) initiates VT (3). At the onset of VT, the marker channel demonstrates a change in the AV conduction pattern. During VT, there is AV dissociation. Markers: TD = tachycardia detected; TS = tachycardia sensing; VS = ventricular sensing.

and ventricular tachyarrhythmias, the first step is to analyze the onset of the tachyarrhythmia. Sinus tachycardia is characterized by a gradual onset, whereas ventricular tachycardia has a sudden onset. The application of the blocks "chamber of origin" and "ventricular electrogram morphology" offers additional information for further differentiation between sinus and ventricular tachycardia. The 'chamber of origin' is used to identify the initiating event at the onset of tachycardia. At the onset of ventricular tachycardia, an intrinsic atrial event usually does not occur between the last conducted

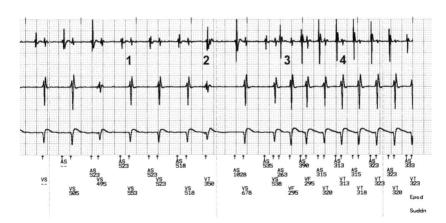

Figure 4.11. Stored electrogram showing atrial tachycardia with consistent 1:1 atrioventricular (AV) conduction. Rhythm strip from top to bottom: atrial, ventricular, and shock electrogram. After six normal conducted ventricular events (1), a ventricular premature beat (2) occurs, which is followed by two normal conducted ventricular events. A premature atrial event (3) initiates an atrial tachycardia with stable 1:1 AV conduction (4). The "chamber of origin" is the atrium and there is no change in the "ventricular electrogram morphology". Markers: AS = atrial sensing; VF = ventricular fibrillation window; VS = ventricular sensing; VT = ventricular tachycardia window; Epsd = initial tachycardia detection met; Suddn = sudden onset; – = no annotation of stored events before detection of tachycardia. (Guidant Prizm DR, model 1861)

sinus beat and the first ventricular ectopic event. On the other hand, an atrial event is present before every ventricular event at the onset of atrial tachycardia (Figure 4.11). It is speculative, but the atrial electrogram should be different when retrograde activation occurs.

The combination of blocks "AV conduction pattern", "chamber of origin", "sudden onset" and "ventricular electrogram morphology" is necessary for challenging tachyarrhythmias with 1:1 AV conduction. Examples are atrial tachycardias with a sudden onset, and sinus or atrial tachycardia with progressive prolongation of the AV conduction.

A Standardized Approach for Electrogram Analysis

For clinical trials, correct electrogram interpretation is important. In a recent study, the overall performance of physicians in electrogram interpretation was similar to the ICD [1, 2, 20]. However, the composition of the misinterpretation was different, which can have a severe impact on the outcome of clinical trials. To improve the accuracy and reproducibility of electrogram analysis, a standardized approach has been developed for a core ICD laboratory (Figure 4.12). We will explain it very briefly here. The electrogram corresponding to the first beat of the tachycardia is labeled "A".

The preceding beat, (usually) the last "normal" conducted sinus beat, is labeled "0". The coupling interval of the premature depolarization initiating the tachycardia (from beat "0" to beat "A") is labeled "V_1". The consecutive intervals of the tachyarrhythmia are numerically sequentially labeled T_1 through T_{12}. The preceding intervals are labeled S_{-1} through S_{-8}. This approach is now under validation and is being used in a large clinical trial [21].

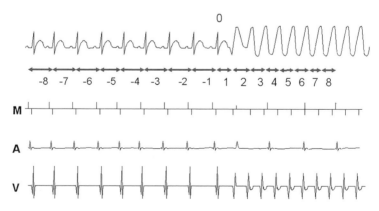

FIGURE 4.12. Schematic approach of the analysis of ventricular tachyarrhythmias. From top to bottom are displayed the surface electrocardiogram (ECG), the marker channel (M), the atrial electrogram (A), and the ventricular electrogram (V). The premature ventricular depolarization initiating the tachyarrhythmia is labeled "A". The preceding interval, the last normal conducted beat, is labeled '0'. The corresponding intervals for analysis are S_{-1} to S_{-8}, V_1, and T_1 to T_{12}.

Preliminary analysis taught us that the most critical step is the definition of the first tachycardia complex. If this is done correctly, further interpetation usually becomes easy when the flow charts as presented in the next chapter are used. It turned out that the core lab was as performant in this way as a team of experienced electrophysiologists.

A Practical Approach to Analyze Electrograms

A first question will always remain whether there is a tachyarrhythmia. Such events can be overlooked as electrograms can be unclear. If so, one should consider that noise (an intracardiac, extracardiac, even extracorporeal source) is interfering with the recording of the electrocardiogram by the device.

If the idea remains present that an arrhythmia is present, one should scan the tracing for the onset. This will reveal whether the arrhythmia starts in the atrium or in the ventricle (if both recordings are available).

The third step is to compare the atrial and ventricular rate, which will reduce the number of possible rhythms.

A fourth step is interpretation of the atrial rhythm (rate, regularity, electrogram), comparing it with the available tracings after conversion, of those available before the arrhythmia. The fifth step does the same with the ventricular rhythm. Critical analysis of the effect of therapy (resetting, changes in rhythm, rate and morphology) will finally elucidate the problem. The next chapter will further describe these practical steps.

It is evident that if all electrogram information is present, a 12-lead electrocardiogram becomes irrelevant for the diagnosis.

References

1. Schaumann A, Brugada J, Capucci A, Appl U. Analysis of stored arrhythmia episodes in implantable cardioverter-defibrillators by 3 electrophysiologists: do we always agree? (abstract). Pacing Clin Electrophysiol 2001;24:612.
2. Theuns DA, Szili-Torok T, Scholten M, Res J, Kimman G, Ruiter J, Jordaens LJ. Stored electrograms in implantable cardioverter defibrillators: agreement upon analysis by electrophysiologists (abstract). Circulation 2002;106:II-322.
3. Intec Systems Inc. Automatic implantable defibrillator clinical investigation. Pittsburgh, 1984.
4. Unterberg C, Stevens J, Vollman D, Hasenfuss G, Buchwald AB. Long-term clinical experience with the EGM width detection criterion for differentiation of supraventricular and ventricular tachycardia in patients with implantable cardioverter defibrillators. Pacing Clin Electrophysiol 2000;23:1611–1617.
5. Swerdlow CD, Mandel WJ, Ziccardi T. Effects of rate and procainamide on electrogram width measured by a tiered-therapy implantable cardioverter-defibrillator (abstract). Pacing Clin Electrophysiol 1996;19:741.

6. Zipes DP. Specific arrhythmias: diagnosis and treatment. In: Braunwald E, editor. Heart disease. A textbook of cardiovascular medicine. Philadelphia: WB Saunders Co, 1997:677–686.

7. Callans DJ, Hook BG, Marchlinski FE. Use of bipolar recordings from patch-patch and rate-sensing leads to distinguish ventricular tachycardias from supraventricular rhythms in patients with implantable cardioverter defibrillators. Pacing Clin Electrophysiol 1991;14:1917–1922.

8. Sarter BH, Hook BG, Callans DJ, Marchlinski FE. Effect of bundle branch block on local electrogram morphology: potential cause of arrhythmia misdiagnosis. Pacing Clin Electrophysiol 1992;15:562.

9. Sarter BH, Hook BG, Callans DJ, Marchlinski FE. Effect of bundle branch block on local electrogram morphologic features: implications for arrhythmia diagnosis by stored electrogram analysis. Am Heart J 1996;131:947–952.

10. Swerdlow CD, Chen PS, Kass RM, Allard JR, Peter CT. Discrimination of ventricular tachycardia from sinus tachycardia and atrial fibrillation in a tiered-therapy cardioverter-defibrillator. J Am Coll Cardiol 1994;23:1342–1355.

11. Kettering K, Dornberger V, Lang R, Vonthein R, Suchalla R, Bosch RF, Mewis C, Eigenberger B, Kuhlkamp V. Enhanced detection criteria in implantable cardioverter defibrillators: sensitivity and specificity of the stability algorithm at different heart rates. Pacing Clin Electrophysiol 2001;24:1325–1333.

12. Neuzner J, Pitschner HF, Schlepper M. Programmable VT detection enhancements in implantable cardioverter defibrillator therapy. Pacing Clin Electrophysiol 1995;18:539–547.

13. Weber M, Bocker D, Bansch D, Brunn J, Castrucci M, Gradaus R, Breithardt G, Block M. Efficacy and safety of the initial use of stability and onset criteria in implantable cardioverter defibrillators. J Cardiovasc Electrophysiol 1999;10:145–153.

14. Hook BG, Callans DJ, Kleiman RB, Flores BT, Marchlinski FE. Implantable cardioverter-defibrillator therapy in the absence of significant symptoms. Rhythm diagnosis and management aided by stored electrogram analysis. Circulation 1993;87:1897–1906.

15. Allessie MA, Bonke FIM. Atrial tachyarrhythmias: basic concepts. In: Mandel WJ, editor. Cardiac arrhythmias. Philadelphia: JB Lippincott Company, 1980:186–207.

16. Saoudi N, Cosio F, Waldo A, Chen SA, Iesaka Y, Lesh M, Saksena S, Salerno J, Schoels W. A classification of atrial flutter and regular atrial tachycardia according to electrophysiological mechanisms and anatomical bases; a Statement from a Joint Expert Group from The Working Group of Arrhythmias of the European Society of Cardiology and the North American Society of Pacing and Electrophysiology. Eur Heart J 2001;22:1162–1182.

17. Morris MM, KenKnight BH, Lang DJ. Detection of atrial arrhythmia for cardiac rhythm management by implantable devices. J Electrocardiol 2000;33(Suppl): 133–139.

18. Wellens HJJ, Bar FW, Vanagt EJ, Brugada P, Farre J. The differentiation between ventricular tachycardia and supraventricular tachycardia with abberant conduction: the value of the 12-lead electrocardiogram. In: Wellens HJJ, Kulbertus HE, editors. What is new in electrocardiography? The Hague: Martinus Nijhoff Pub., 1981:184–199.

19. Saeed M, Link MS, Mahapatra S, Mouded M, Tzeng D, Jung V, Contreras R, Swygman C, Homoud M, Estes NA, 3rd, Wang PJ. Analysis of intracardiac electrograms showing monomorphic ventricular tachycardia in patients with implantable cardioverter-defibrillators. Am J Cardiol 2000;85:580–587.

20. Kim MH, Bruckman D, Sticherling C, Pelosi F, Knight BP, Oral H, Morady F, Strick-berger A. The utility of dual-chamber electrogram recordings for the diagnosis of clinical tachycardias (abstract). J Am Coll Cardiol 2002;39(Suppl 1):78A.

21. Brouwer IA, Zock PL, Wever EF, Hauer RN, Camm AJ, Bocker D, Otto-Terlouw P, Katan MB, Schouten EG. Rationale and design of a randomised controlled clinical trial on supplemental intake of n-3 fatty acids and incidence of cardiac arrhythmia: SOFA. Eur J Clin Nutr 2003;57:1323–1330.

5
A Practical Approach to Analyze Stored Electrograms

Summary

A step-wise logical approach is presented both for devices with and without atrial information. The presented flow charts can help to interpret rhythm strips, but keep their limitations, certainly for single chamber devices.

Rhythms detected by the ICD may represent either a tachyarrhythmia, which can be atrial or ventricular, or oversensing of electrical signals (Figure 5.1). The first step in the analysis of stored electrograms is to determine whether a true tachyarrhythmia is present (Figure 5.2).

In the absence of a true tachyarrhythmia, inappropriate therapy is mainly caused by oversensing of intracardiac or extracardiac signals. Intracardiac signals that can cause oversensing include P, R, or T waves (Figure 5.3). Ventricular oversensing of intracardiac signals results in more than one detected ventricular activitiy per cardiac cycle. Dependent on the cardiac cycle, ventricular oversensing can result in inappropriate detection of ventricular tachyarrhythmias either in the tachycardia detection zone or in the fibrillation detection zone. Oversensing of intracardiac signals can be recognized by characteristics alternation of intervals and electrogram morphology separated by isoelectric baseline. Extracardiac signals include electromagnetic interference, signals generated by lead or connector problems, and myopotentials. The hallmark of oversensing of extracardiac signals is the replacement of the isoelectric baseline with high-frequency noise.

If the device is triggered by a true tachyarrhythmia, the investigator has to determine if the initial detected rhythm is a ventricular tachyarrhythmia or an atrial tachyarrhythmia. The second step in the analysis of stored electrograms is to determine the onset of the tachyarrhythmia. Figure 5.4 shows the second step of the analysis for single-chamber and dual-chamber electrograms.

The ventricular electrogram and the marker channel are used to determine the onset of the tachyarrhythmia. The first step is to determine the last normal conducted beat followed by the first beat of the tachyarrhythmia. In the marker channel, the first beat of the tachyarrhythmia is often labeled as "TS", preceded by a normal beat labeled as "VS". The ventricular electrogram can be used to confirm the onset of a ventricular tachyarrhythmia. The tachyarrhythmia is classified as ventricular if the morphology during tachyarrhythmia is distinctly different from the baseline rhythm (Figures 5.5 and 5.6).

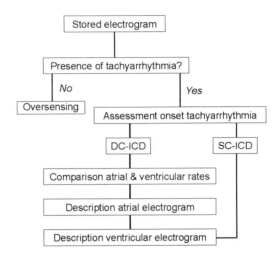

FIGURE 5.1. Steps in a practical approach to analyze stored electrograms. DC: dual chanber ICD; SC: single chamber ICD.

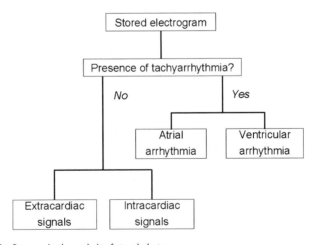

FIGURE 5.2. The first step in the analysis of stored electrograms.

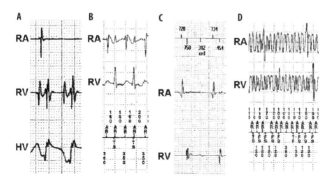

FIGURE 5.3. Oversensing of intracardiac signals which can result in inappropriate detection of ventricular tachyarrhythmias. Panel A shows R-wave double counting during monomorphic ventricular tachycardia. B shows oversensing of R-wave on the atrial bipolar electrogram (far-field R-wave oversensing). C shows T-wave oversensing on the ventricular bipolar electrogram. D shows electromagnetic interference on the atrial and ventricular electrogram. HV: (high voltage) far-field ventricular electrogram; RA = right atrial electrogram; RV: near-field ventricular electrogram.

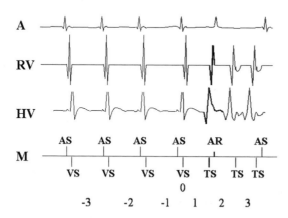

FIGURE 5.4. Assessment of the onset of tachyarrhythmia. From top to bottom: A = atrial electrogram; RV = near-field ventricular electrogram; HV = (high voltage) far-field ventricular electrogram; M = marker channel. Markers: AR = atrial refractory sense; AS = atrial sense; TS = tachycardia sense; VS = ventricular sense.

Stored Electrograms in Single-chamber Devices

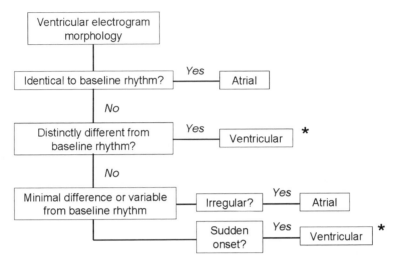

FIGURE 5.5. Approach for analysis of stored electrograms in single-chamber devices.
* aberrancy cannot be excluded

Stored Electrograms in Dual-chamber Devices

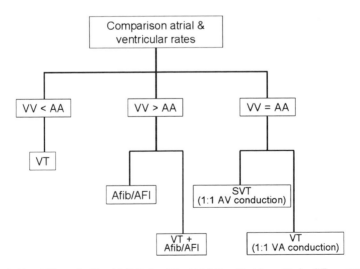

FIGURE 5.6. AA: atrial intervals; AF: atrial fibrillation; AFL: atrial flutter; AV: atrio-ventricular; SVT: supraventricular tachycardia; VA: ventriculo-atrial; VT: ventricular tachycardia; VV: ventricular intervals.

6
Clinical Case Studies

Early Devices

Case 1 Out-of-Hospital Cardiac Arrest after ICD Implantation

Patient: 42-year-old male with familial dilated cardiomyopathy and diabetes, left ventricular ejection fraction 19%, NYHA functional class II, with frequent ventricular premature beats.

Index arrhythmia: ventricular fibrillation.

Problem: admission after out-of-hospital cardiac arrest with external defibrillation by the emergency squad.

ICD pulse generator: Ventak 1625 with an Endotak 072 lead (Guidant/CPI, USA).

Tachycardia settings
Detection: VT = 180/min.
Duration: 2, 5 s.
COMMITTED.

Bradycardia settings
VVI 40 bpm.

Electrogram (*See* Figure 6.1a)

Electrogram interpretation
Wide band ventricular electrogram, obtained via standard electrocardiographer, coupled to the programming wand. The sequence shows six consecutive arrhythmias (recognized as VT when upward spikes are displayed). Only the first five are shocked (downward spikes, numbered from 1 to 5). The first event is polymorphic VT degenerating to VF. The initial rhythm is faster than 180 bpm. The complexes are illegible after the shocks because of a polarization effect.
Fortunately, the rescue squad arrived after this sequence.

Diagnosis: For the first event: polymorphic VT, degenerating to VF.

Action: defibrillation; metoprolol IV; the patient was put on the emergency list for heart transplantation.

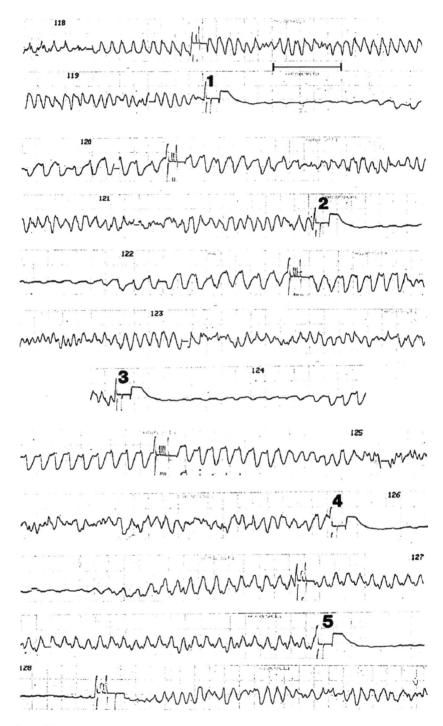

FIGURE 6.1a.

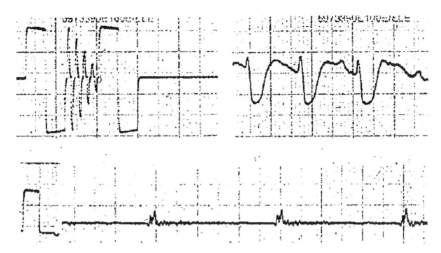

FIGURE 6.1b.

Online electrograms (*See* Figure 6.1b)

From top to bottom: surface electrocardiogram obtained by coupling a standard ECG machine to the programming wand and a bipolar (near-field) intracardiac ventricular electrogram. The latter was obtained at the time of ICD removal, during heart transplantation.

Diagnosis: sinus rhythm, with intraventricular conduction delay (the QRS width is at least 240 ms). The intracardiac amplitude is very small (less than 0.5 mV). The morphology of the available wide band electrogram in sinus rhythm suggests that arrhythmias 2, 3, and 4 might have been fast conducted supraventricular rhythm.

Case 2 Multiple Morphologies in a Single Episode

Patient: 49-year-old man with old infarction, left ventricular ejection fraction 0.28, no evident heart failure, and history of atrial flutter.

Index arrhythmia: sustained monomorphic ventricular tachycardia, cycle length 290 ms. Remained inducible on sotalol, what was continued (1993).

Complaint: frequent shocks within the first six months.

Electrogram

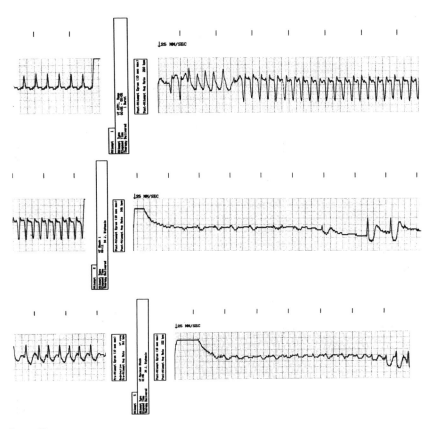

FIGURE 6.2.

ICD pulse generator: Ventak 1715 (CPI, later Guidant, USA). Shock delivered between RV coil and subcutaneous array with SVC coil – DFT 15 J.

Electrogram interpretation

Shock-lead electrograms. In the first strip ATP (burst) is delivered for a narrow QRS complex tachycardia with TCL of 360 ms, resulting in a polymorphic wide QRS tachycardia, ending in a regular wide QRS complex tachycardia with TCL of 240 ms. In the second strip, this wide QRS complex tachycardia is treated with a 34 J shock, resulting in an illegible rhythm strip, transitioning to an irregular, narrow complex rhythm, which again is given a biphasic 34 J shocked in strip 3, resulting in no definite electrogram changes, except for repolarization disturbances.

Diagnosis: the initiating arrhythmia is atrial flutter with 2:1 atrioventricular conduction; the final strip shows atrial fibrillation. With the available information no definite diagnosis can be made for the wide QRS tachycardia in strips 1 and 2.

Single Chamber Devices

Case 3 A Diverted Defibrillator Shock

Patient: 54-year-old female with ischemic heart disease, old anterior wall myocardial infarction.

Index arrhythmia: out-of-hospital arrest, ventricular fibrillation.

Observation: diverted defibrillator shock.

Electrogram

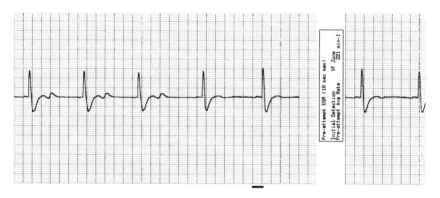

Figure 6.3a. Stored wide-band (shock) electrogram.

ICD pulse generator: Ventak Mini IV (Guidant Inc, St Paul, MN, USA).

Tachycardia settings
Detection: VF = 270 ms; VT = 315 ms.
Discrimination: onset = 16%; stability = 30 ms.
Therapy: VF = shock; VT = antitachycardia pacing and cardioversion.

Bradycardia settings
Mode: VVI 40 bpm.

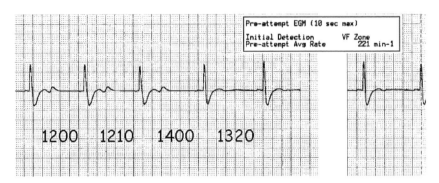

FIGURE **6.3b.** The text box states an initial detection in the ventricular fibrillation zone, rate 221 bpm. Real measurements of the RR interval.

Electrogram interpretation (*See* Figure 6.3b)

Interpretation

1. *Presence of tachyarrhythmia?*: No.
2. *Presence of high-frequency noise on isoelectric baseline?*: No.
3. *Description of the shock electrogram*: The morphology of the ventricular activity is consistent with a cycle length of ≈1200 ms and a stability of ≈10 ms (Electrogram above). Despite this slow ventricular rhythm, ventricular fibrillation is detected as mentioned in the text box. The electrogram is therefore not helpful. Additional information is required, which is provided by the RR interval table (see the next figure).
4. *Analysis of the RR interval table*: This table confirms that normally conducted beats are present (cycle length ≈1200 ms). However, signals in the ventricular fibrillation detection zone are sensed as well with a cycle length of <270 ms. The diverted shock therapy occurred in the absence of a true tachyarrhythmia because physiological or non-physiological signals are oversensed and detected as an arrhythmia.
5. *Assessment of the origin of oversensed signals*: The oversensed signals can be due to lead or connector problem, or oversensing of myopotentials. Oversensing due to lead or connector problems may be limited to the rate-sensing electrode. Measurement of pacing-lead impedance was normal. During provocation tests, no oversensing was registered. (*See* Figure 6.3c)

Episode 91	R-R Intervals								

	Date 07-MAR-2005		Time 08:17			Type Spontaneous			
Onset	1188 --	1150 --	1199 --	1199 --	1199 --	1199 --	1199 --	842 --	148 VF	197 VF
	178 VF	617 VS	141 VF	266 VF	211 VF	596 VS	152 VF	160 VF		
Initial Detection	232 VF	143 VF	160 VF	463 VS	141 VF	156 VF	291 VT	156 VF	564 VS	143 VF
	223 VF									
Attempt 1 VF Shk1	240 VF Chrg	568 VS Chrg	162 VF Chrg	273 VF Chrg	303 VT Chrg	922 VS Chrg	172 VF Chrg	686 VS Chrg	383 VS Chrg	279 VT Chrg
	1199 VP Chrg	1197 VS Chrg	1152 VS Chrg	496 --	717 VS	1240 VS	1215 VS	1199 --		
Redetection	1199 VP	1199 VP	1199 VP	1199 VP	1199 VP	1199 VP	1199 VP	1199 VP		

End of Episode

FIGURE 6.3c.

Diagnosis: sinus rhythm with oversensing of extracardiac physiological signals, probably myopotentials.

Action: reprogrammation of ventricular sensitivity. This solved the problem, which never occurred again over the next five years.

Case 4 Hypokalemia, Late After Infarction

Patient: 54-year-old female with ischemic heart disease, old anterior wall myocardial infarction.

Index arrhythmia: out-of-hospital arrest, ventricular fibrillation.

Complaint: admission one month after implantation because of several consecutive shocks. After defibrillator implantation, pharmacological treatment consisted of 80 mg furosemide, 250 μg digoxine, 10 mg fosinopril, and 25 mg spironolacton, in combination with 200 mg amiodarone.

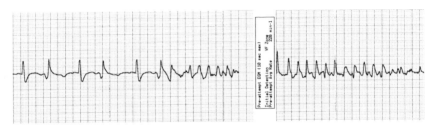

FIGURE 6.4a.

ICD pulse generator: Ventak Mini IV (Guidant Inc, St Paul, MN, USA).

Tachycardia settings
Detection: VF = 270 ms; VT = 315 ms.
Discrimination: onset = 16%; stability = 30 ms.
Therapy: VF = shock; VT = antitachycardia pacing and cardioversion.

Bradycardia settings
Mode: VVI 40 bpm.

Electrogram interpretation (*See* Figure 6.4b)

1. *Presence of tachyarrhythmia?*: Yes.
2. *Assessment of the onset of the tachyarrhythmia triggering device therapy*: the stored bipolar shock electrogram demonstrates ventricular premature beats (*) during sinus rhythm, in bigeminy. After a third ventricular premature beat, a fast polymorphic ventricular tachycardia (arrow) is initiated.

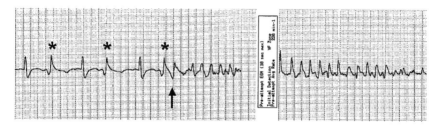

FIGURE 6.4b. Stored bipolar shock electrogram.

3. *Characteristics of the ventricular electrogram during the tachyarrhythmia*: the morphology of the ventricular activity is polymorphic during tachycardia. The morphology of the shock electrogram during tachycardia changed as compared to the baseline rhythm. The tachycardia has a ventricular cycle length of ≈250 ms, with a stability of ≈10 ms.

Diagnosis: ventricular bigeminy, late coupled ventricular premature beat, inducing polymorphic ventricular tachycardia.

Action: Analysis of electrolytes; potassium was 2.4 mg/L; surface ECG.

Surface ECG

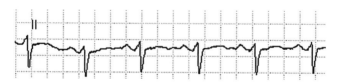

FIGURE 6.4c. The electrocardiogram after adjustment of electrolytes, and after correction of polypharmacia. Lead II still shows a QT interval of 462 ms, with an RR interval of 723 ms and a QTc of 501 ms.

Case 5 Assessment After Syncope

Patient: 80-year-old male with ischemic heart disease, coronary artery bypass grafting, left ventricular ejection fraction <0.35, and permanent atrial fibrillation.

Index arrhythmia: non-sustained ventricular tachycardias.

Complaint: Syncope.

Electrogram (Two continuous strips are shown).

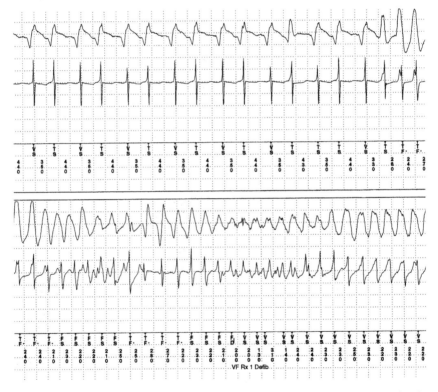

FIGURE 6.5a. From top to bottom: far-field ventricular electrogram, near-field ventricular electrogram, and marker channel. Markers: FD = fibrillation detected; FS = fibrillation sensing; TF: fast tachycardia sensing; TS = tachycardia sensing.

ICD pulse generator: Gem VR 7221 (Medtronic Inc, Minneapolis, MN, USA).

Tachycardia settings
Detection: VF = 300 ms; fast VT via VF = 260 ms; VT = 370 ms.

Discrimination: stability = 30 ms.

Therapy: VF = shock; fast VT and VT = antitachycardia pacing and cardioversion.

Bradycardia settings

Mode: VVIR 60–120 bpm.

Electrogram interpretation

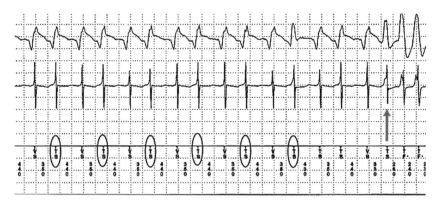

FIGURE 6.5b.

1. *Presence of tachyarrhythmia?*: Yes.
2. *Assessment of the onset of the tachyarrhythmia triggering device therapy*: the stored ventricular electrogram demonstrates bigeminy during baseline rhythm (the alternation of VS and TS in the marker channel). After a ventricular premature beat (arrow), a fast polymorphic ventricular tachycardia is initiated.

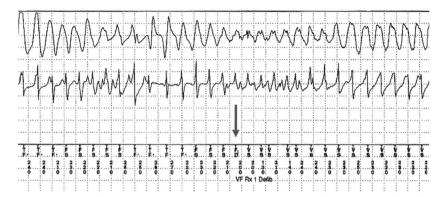

FIGURE 6.5c.

3. *Characteristics of the ventricular electrogram during the tachyarrhythmia*: the morphology of the ventricular activity is polymorphic during tachycardia. The morphology of both ventricular electrograms during tachycardia changed as compared to the baseline rhythm. The tachycardia has a ventricular cycle length of ≈ 230 ms, with a stability of ≈ 10 ms.

Diagnosis: ventricular bigeminy, late coupled ventricular premature beat, inducing polymorphic ventricular tachycardia, qualifying for VF detection (FD) by the device.

Case 6 An Uncommon Initiation of an Arrhythmia

Patient: 66-year-old male with ischemic heart disease, congestive heart failure, left ventricular ejection fraction 0.30, left bundle branch block (QRS width 142 ms) and permanent atrial fibrillation. The patient was listed for cardiac transplantation.

Index arrhythmia: sustained monomorphic ventricular tachycardias, cycle length 300 ms.

Complaint: Syncope and shock therapy by the ICD.

Electrogram

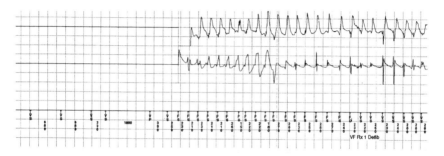

FIGURE 6.6a. From top to bottom: far-field ventricular electrogram, near-field ventricular electrogram, and marker channel. Markers: FD = fibrillation detected; FS = fibrillation sensing; VP = ventricular pace; VS = ventricular sense.

ICD pulse generator: Gem 7227 VR (Medtronic Inc, Minneapolis, MN, USA).

Tachycardia settings
Detection: VF = 290 ms; VT = 340 ms.
Discrimination: stability = 30 ms.
Therapy: VF = shock; VT = antitachycardia pacing and cardioversion.

Bradycardia settings
Mode: VVIR 60–120 bpm.

Electrogram interpretation (*See* Figure 6.6b)

1. *Presence of tachyarrhythmia?*: Yes.
2. *Assessment of the onset of the tachyarrhythmia triggering the device*: A second premature beat initiates a fast tachyarrhythmia.

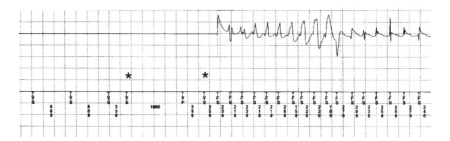

FIGURE 6.6b.

3. *Characteristics of the ventricular electrogram during the tachyarrhythmia*: the morphology of the ventricular activity is variable in both ventricular electrograms. The morphology cannot be compared to the baseline rhythm, as no electrogram was stored before arrhythmia onset. Additional information can be provided by the stored electrogram after delivered device therapy. The ventricular rhythm has a cycle length of ≈225 ms, with a stability of ≈30 ms.

4. *Characteristics of the ventricular electrogram after device therapy*: the morphology of the ventricular activity after device therapy changed as compared to morphology during the tachyarrhythmia (Figure 6.6c).

Diagnosis: fast polymorphic ventricular tachycardia induced by a ventricular premature beat in a short-long-short sequence.

Action: the lower rate of the pacemaker can be increased, but this may increase the percentage of right ventricular pacing.

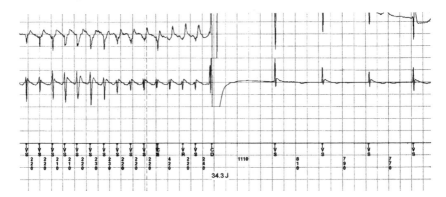

FIGURE 6.6c. From top to bottom: far-field ventricular electrogram, near-field ventricular electrogram, and marker channel. Markers: CD = charge delivered; CE = charge end; VR = ventricular refractory; VS = ventricular sense.

Case 7 A Patient with Congenital Heart Disease and Therapies for a Short Arrhythmia

Patient: 29-year-old male with surgically corrected complex congenital heart disease (double outlet right ventricle; malposition of the great arteries, VSD, and coarctation), left ventricular dysfunction, and superior vena cava syndrome, uses salbutamol inhalator because he is asthmatic. QRS width 170 ms.

Index arrhythmia: sustained monomorphic ventricular tachycardia, cycle length 490 ms.

Complaint: recurrent palpitations, syncopal, wants to drive.

Electrogram (Three continuous strips).

ICD pulse generator: Maximo VR 7232 (Medtronic Inc, Minneapolis, MN, USA). Epicardiac sensing electrodes and 6721 defibrillator patch.

Tachycardia settings
Detection: VF = 280 ms; fast VT = 240 ms; VT = 400 ms.
Discrimination: stability = 30 ms; onset = 84%.
Therapy: VF = shock; fast VT = antitachycardia pacing and shock; VT = antitachycardia pacing.

Bradycardia settings
Mode: VVI 40 bpm; all fancy features off.

Electrogram interpretation (*See* Figure 6.7a)

1. *Presence of tachycardia:* yes.
2. *Description of the onset:* described by the device in the first strip as "gradual", which is not correct, when the intervals are considered.
3. *Characteristics of the ventricular electrogram during the tachyarrhythmia:* the morphology of the FF and NF ventricular activity is similar and as wide as the complexes after spontaneous slowing. Only a little notch in the last part of the QRS in the NF electrogram suggests a different activation, which can be as easily explained as aberrancy.
4. *Additional criteria and effect of therapy:* the tachycardia CL varies between 230 and 240 ms in the first strip, before the slowing and the criteria for VF are met, triggering a shock. This does not affect the rhythm, varying between 370 and 390 ms in the second tracing, triggering ATP, once more not altering the QRS pattern.

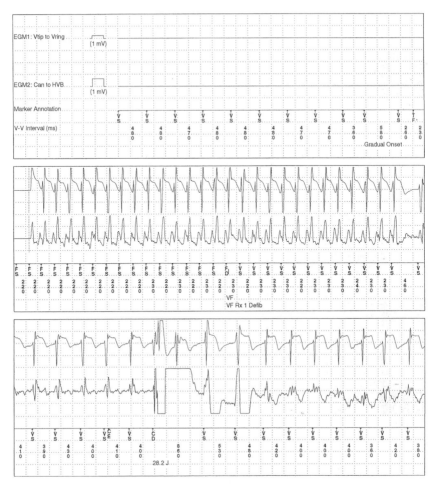

FIGURE 6.7a. First strip: Markers: CD = charge delivered; CE = charge end; FD = fibrillation detected; FS = fibrillation sensing; TF = sense in fast VT window; VS = ventricular sense. Second and third strip: From top to bottom: near field, wide-band ventricular electrogram and markers.

Diagnosis: uncertain – supraventricular tachycardia with wide QRS complexes remains possible (see figure 6.7b). Former electrograms showed a more distinctive tachycardia pattern. The tachogram (not shown, but very gradual) and the salbutamol use suggest atrial tachycardia.

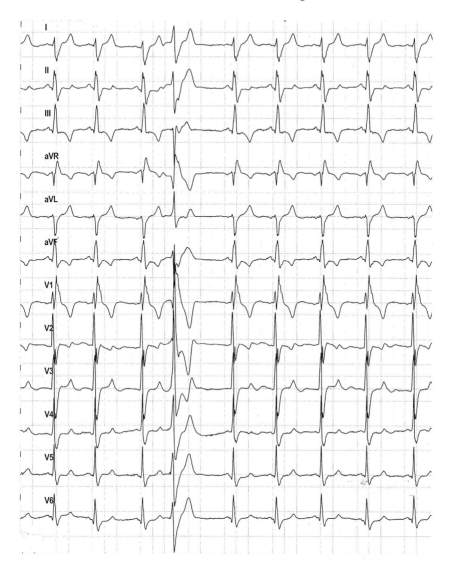

Figure 6.7b.

Actions: Increase the number of intervals before detection or confirmation.

Case 8 An Arrhythmia Detected by Remote Monitoring

Patient: 54-year-old male, with mitral valve prothesis, coronary artery disease (PTCA with stent 2 years ago), COPD, heart failure, and persistent atrial fibrillation. ICD at age 50, recent replacement with a home-monitoring unit.

Index arrhythmia: non-sustained ventricular tachycardia.

Complaint: none.

Electrogram (as transmitted by GSM and Internet).

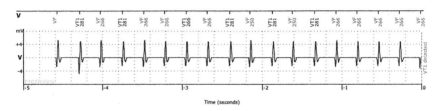

FIGURE 6.8a. Ventricular intervals (Grey for VF, Black for VT1); ventricular bipolar electrogram.

ICD pulse generator: Lumos VRT (Biotronik, Erlangen Germany)

Tachycardia settings
Detection: VF = 270 ms; VT1 = 400 ms; no VT2).
Discrimination: onset = 15%; stability = 40 ms.
Therapy: VF = shock; VT = antitachycardia pacing (burst).

Bradycardia settings Mode: VVI 50 bpm.

Electrogram Interpretation

1. *Tachycardia*: present (cycle length 266 ms at the end; some irregularity in the beginning with a longer coupling of 281 ms, bringing the rhythm in the VT zone).
2. *Comparison between atrial and ventricular rate*: not possible.
3. *Assessment of the onset of the tachyarrhythmia*: not transmitted.
4. *Characteristics of the ventricular electrogram during the tachyarrhythmia*: the morphology of the ventricular activity is always the same; it has a width of 0.09 s.

5. The *atrioventricular relationship* is unclear (no atrial channel).
6. *Therapy* is not displayed, but the transmission says that ATP was given.

Electrogram at subsequent consultation

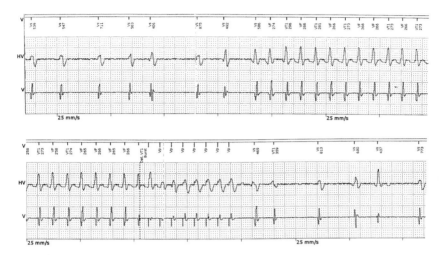

FIGURE 6.8b. From top to bottom: ventricular marker channel with ventricular intervals; ventricular wide-band and bipolar electrograms (respectively HV and V). VF = ventricular fibrillation; VT1 = ventricular tachycardia; VP = ventricular pacing; VS = ventricular sensing.

1. *Tachycardia*: confirmed.
2. *Assessment of the onset of the tachyarrhythmia*: the baseline rhythm is probably atrial fibrillation. After a rather long pause a VPB is followed by a regular tachycardia with a different, wide QRS morphology and a cycle length as was transmitted in the former electrogram.
3. The atrioventricular relationship remains unclear (see above).
4. ATP (7 pulses) restores the initial rhythm, interrupted by a ventricular premature beat.

Diagnosis: atrial fibrillation, followed by sustained monomorphic ventricular tachycardia.

Actions: none. The home monitoring was continued.

Dual Chamber Devices

Case 9 A Neonate with an ICD and LQT3

Patient: neonate boy with drug refractory ventricular arrhythmias turning out to be long QT syndrome (LQT3).

Index arrhythmia: ventricular fibrillation, out-of-hospital cardiac arrest.

Complaint: 7 months after implantation parents observed a shock.

Electrogram

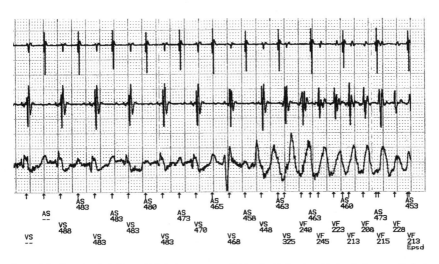

Figure 6.9a. From top to bottom: atrial electrogram, near-field and wide-band ventricular electrogram. Markers: AS = atrial sensing; VF = ventricular fibrillation; VS = ventricular sensing.

ICD pulse generator: Prizm DR 1853 HE (Guidant Inc, St Paul, MN, USA); epicardial sense/pace leads and epicardial defibrillation patch.

Tachycardia settings
Detection: VF = 285 ms.
Therapy: VF = shock.

Bradycardia settings
Mode: AAI 70 bpm.

Electrogram interpretation

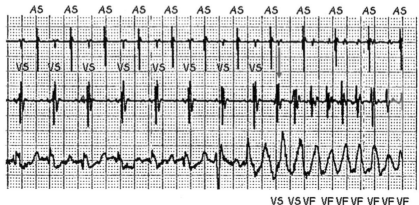

FIGURE 6.9b.

1. The first step in electrogram interpretation is the comparison between atrial and ventricular rate, which results in rate branch VV < AA.
2. The second step is a description of the atrial rhythm. The atrial electrogram shows large as well as small deflections. The small deflection represents far-field sensing of the ventricular activity. The large deflection represents an atrial rhythm with a cycle length ≈470 ms with a consistent morphology. The atrial electrogram demonstrates sinus tachycardia.
3. The third step is the assessment of the onset of the tachyarrhythmia triggering device therapy. The ventricular and shock electrogram demonstrate normal conducted beats during sinus tachycardia. After a ventricular premature beat (arrow), a tachyarrhythmia is initiated, which is not in the VF zone for the first two beats.
4. Finally, we describe the characteristics of the ventricular electrogram during the tachyarrhythmia. The morphology of the ventricular and shock electrogram during tachycardia changed as compared to the baseline rhythm. The tachycardia has a ventricular cycle length of ≈ 220 ms, with a stability of ≈ 15 ms. The atrial rate is not affected during the tachyarrhythmia, and there is no consistent atrioventricular relation.

Diagnosis: polymorphic ventricular tachycardia. This will degenerate immediately into ventricular fibrillation.

Further actions: antiarrhythmic drug therapy with flecainide.

Case 10 Tachycardia after Antiarrhythmic Drugs

Patient: neonate at age of 3 years.

Index arrhythmia: out-of-hospital cardiac arrest, ventricular fibrillation due to LQT3.

Complaint: recurrent shocks.

Electrogram

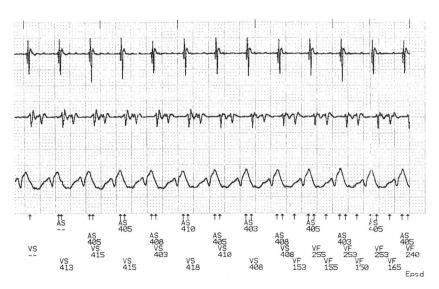

FIGURE 6.10a. From top to bottom: atrial electrogram, near-field and wide-band ventricular electrogram, and markers. Markers: AS = atrial sensing; Epsd = episode; VF = ventricular fibrillation; VS = ventricular sensing.

ICD pulse generator: Prizm DR 1853 HE (Guidant Inc, St Paul, MN, USA); epicardial sense/pace leads and epicardial defibrillation patch.

Tachycardia settings
Detection: VF = 285 ms.
Therapy: VF = shock.

Bradycardia settings
Mode: AAI 70 bpm.

Electrogram interpretation

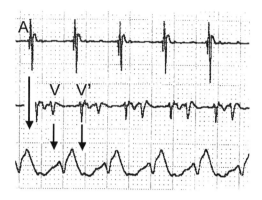

FIGURE 6.10b. From top to bottom: atrial electrogram (A), near-field and wide-band ventricular electrogram (splitted in V and V').

1. *Comparison between atrial and ventricular rate*: rate branch VV = AA.
2. *Description of the atrial rhythm*: the atrial electrogram shows a fast atrial rhythm with cycle length ≈415 ms with a consistent atrial morphology. The atrial electrogram demonstrates sinus tachycardia.

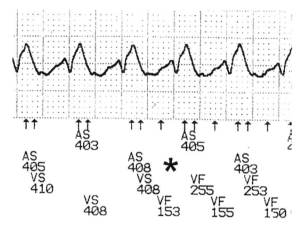

FIGURE 6.10c. Wide-band electrogram and marker channel. Markers: AS = atrial sensing; Epsd = episode; VF = ventricular fibrillation; VS = ventricular sensing.

3. *Assessment of the onset of the tachyarrhythmia triggering device therapy*: the marker channel demonstrates sensed activations in the ventricular fibrillation window (*). These sensed activations have a consistent sequence of a short (155 ms) and a long interval (250 ms) for each ventricular depolarization.

4. *Characteristics of the ventricular electrogram during the tachyarrhythmia*: the morphology of the ventricular and shock electrogram during tachycardia is stable with a consistent atrioventricular relation. The PR (A-V) interval measured between the electrograms is 180 ms; the split bipolar ventricular and wide band ventricular electrogram width measure ≈230 ms! The tachycardia has a ventricular cycle length of ≈415 ms.

Diagnosis: double counting of ventricular depolarization due to increased dosage of flecainide as antiarrhythmic drug treatment.

Further action: lower dose of flecainide.

Case 11 Changes in the Electrogram Morphology During Tachycardia

Patient: 73-year-old male with ischemic heart disease, paroxysmal atrial fibrillation.

Index arrhythmia: ventricular fibrillation, cardiac arrest.

Complaint: shock.

Electrogram

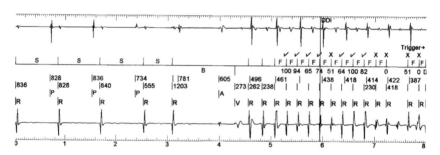

Figure 6.11a. From top to bottom: atrial electrogram, marker channel, and ventricular electrogram. Markers: A = atrial pacing; B = bradycardia window; F = ventricular fibrillation window; P = atrial sense; R = ventricular sense; S = sinus window; TS = tachycardia sensing; V = ventricular pacing.

ICD pulse generator: Atlas DR 243 (St Jude Medical, Sylmar, CA, USA).

Tachycardia settings

Detection: VF = 300 ms; fast VT via VF = 270 ms; VT = 430 ms.
Discrimination: onset 16%; stability = 30 ms; morphology discrimination ON.
Therapy: VF = shock; fast VT and VT = antitachycardia pacing and cardioversion.

Bradycardia settings
Mode: DDI 50 bpm.
AV = 275 ms.

Electrogram interpretation

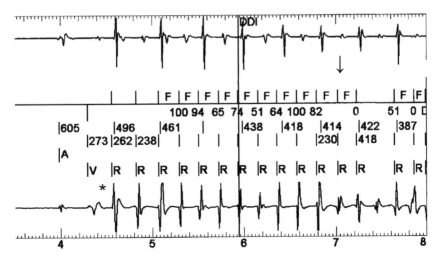

Figure 6.11b.

1. *Presence of tachyarrhythmia?*: Yes.
2. *Assessment of the onset of the tachyarrhythmia triggering the device*: the first VV interval in the tachycardia detection zone (*) indicates the onset of the tachyarrhythmia.
3. *Comparison between atrial and ventricular rate*: rate branch VV < AA.
4. *Description of the atrial rhythm*: the atrial electrogram shows large as well as small deflections. The small deflection represents far-field oversensing of the ventricular activity. The large deflection represents an atrial rhythm, cycle length ≈420 ms, with a consistent morphology. The atrial electrogram demonstrates sinus tachycardia.
5. *Characteristics of the ventricular electrogram during the tachyarrhythmia*: the morphology of the ventricular activity is initially consistent during tachycardia. After 11 beats, the morphology is changing (arrow). The atrioventricular conduction pattern can be assessed from the marker channel. During the tachycardia, the marker channel demonstrates a consistent atrioventricular relationship of ≈160 ms. The tachycardia has a ventricular cycle length of ≈360 ms, with a stability of ≈10 ms.

Diagnosis: appropriate detection of fast polymorphic ventricular tachycardia.

Action: reprogrammation of the bradycardia settings, increase of the lower rate and decrease of the AV interval.

Case 12 A Shock at Washing Day

Patient: 46-year-old male with corrected Fallot's tetralogy.

Index arrhythmia: sustained monomorphic ventricular tachycardia.

Complaint: Shock when doing the laundry.

Electrogram

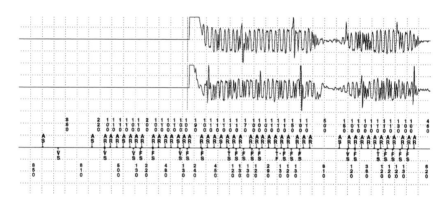

FIGURE **6.12a.** From top to bottom: atrial electrogram, ventricular electrogram, and marker channel. Markers: AR = atrial refractory sense; AS = atrial sense; TF = tachycardia sense (fast ventricular tachycardia window); TS = tachycardia sense (ventricular tachycardia window); VF = ventricular fibrillation sense; VS = ventricular sense.

ICD pulse generator: Marquis DR 7274 (Medtronic Inc, Minneapolis, MN, USA).

Tachycardia settings
Detection: VF = 300 ms; fast VT via VF = 270 ms; VT = 430 ms.
Discrimination: stability = 40 ms; PR Logic ON.
Therapy: VF = shock; fast VT and VT = antitachycardia pacing and cardioversion.

Bradycardia settings
Mode: DDD 70–120 bpm.
Mode switch = ON.
AV = 110 ms.

Electrogram interpretation

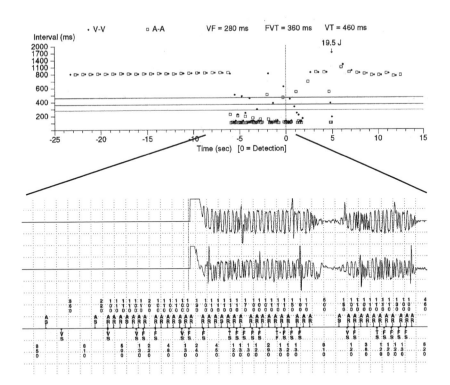

FIGURE 6.12b.

1. *Presence of tachyarrhythmia?*: No.
2. *Presence of high-frequency noise on isoelectric baseline?*: Yes.
3. *Interval plot*: the interval versus time plot shows AA intervals and VV intervals with cycle length of 100–150 ms. These short intervals are an indication of high-frequency noise due to non-physiological signals.
4. *Description of the atrial and ventricular electrogram*: the atrial and ventricular electrograms show large as well as sinusoidal deflections. The large deflections represent the baseline rhythm, cycle length ≈850 ms. The sinusoidal deflections demonstrate high-frequency noise due to electromagnetic interference.

Diagnosis: external electromagnetic interference.

Action: instructions for the patient to avoid sources of electromagnetic interference. Grounding of the washing machine.

Case 13 Regular Tachycardia, 150 Beats Per Minute

Patient: 67-year-old male with ischemic heart disease, coronary artery bypass grafting.

Index arrhythmia: sustained monomorphic ventricular tachycardia.

Complaint: palpitations.

Electrogram

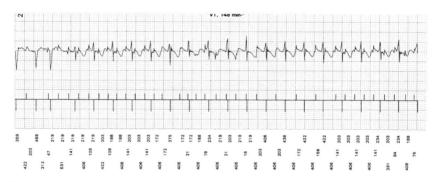

FIGURE 6.13a. From top to bottom: wide-band electrogram, markers, and device activity channel.

ICD pulse generator: Defender IV DR 612 (ELA Medical, Le Plessis, France).

Tachycardia settings
Detection: VF = 300 ms; fast VT via VF = 270 ms; VT = 430 ms.
Discrimination: stability = 40 ms; PR Logic ON.
Therapy: VF = shock; fast VT and VT = antitachycardia pacing and cardioversion.

Bradycardia settings
Mode: DDD 70–120 bpm.
Mode switch = ON.
AV = 110 ms.

Electrogram interpretation

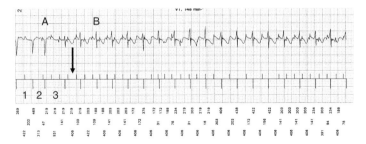

FIGURE 6.13b.

1. *Presence of tachyarrhythmia?*: Yes.
2. *Assessment of the onset of the tachyarrhythmia triggering the device*: the first three VV intervals of the device activity channel are irregular (1, 2, and 3). After these intervals, the device activity channel demonstrates a stable ventricular rhythm (arrow).
3. *Comparison between atrial and ventricular rate*: rate branch VV > AA.
4. *Description of the atrial rhythm*: the wide-band electrogram shows small deflections, which represent the atrial activity. The device activity channel confirms the atrial activity with cycle length ≈200 ms. The device activity channel also shows longer atrial intervals. These intervals can be explained by the presence of ventriculoatrial crossblanking of the device. The morphology of the atrial activity is consistent. The atrial rhythm can either be atrial fibrillation or atrial flutter.
5. *Characteristics of the ventricular electrogram during the tachyarrhythmia*: the morphology of the ventricular activity is consistent during tachycardia. The morphology of the ventricular activity during tachycardia (A) changed as compared to the baseline rhythm (B). The tachycardia has a ventricular cycle length of ≈406 ms, with a stability <10 ms.
6. *Atrioventricular relationship*: the atrioventricular conduction pattern can be assessed from the device activity channel. During tachycardia, the device activity channel demonstrates absence of a consistent atrioventricular relationship, which favors the presence of a ventricular tachycardia. Additional information to assess the presence of a ventricular tachycardia during atrial fibrillation or atrial flutter is provided by the electrogram after device therapy.
7. *Characteristics of the ventricular electrogram after therapy*: the morphology of the ventricular activity after antitachycardia pacing is consistent (electrogram below). The morphology of the ventricular activity is similar to the first three VV intervals in the first electrogram.

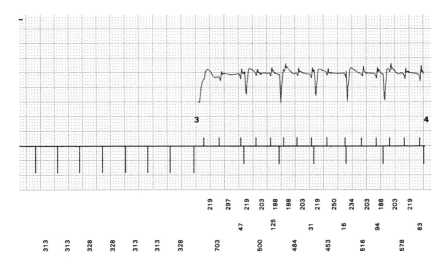

FIGURE 6.13c. From top to bottom: wide-band electrogram, markers, and device activity channel.

Diagnosis: ventricular tachycardia during atrial fibrillation or atrial flutter.

Action: no action required.

Case 14 Tiny Spikes on the Wide Band Electrogram

Patient: 73-year-old male with ischemic heart disease, coronary artery bypass grafting, left ventricular ejection fraction 32%.

Index arrhythmia: out-of-hospital arrest, ventricular fibrillation.

Complaint: shock.

Electrogram

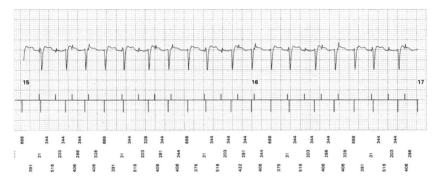

Figure 6.14a. From top to bottom: wide-band electrogram, markers, and device activity channel.

ICD pulse generator: Defender IV DR 612 (ELA Medical, Le Plessis, France).

Tachycardia settings
Detection: VF = 300 ms; VT = 405 ms.
Discrimination: onset = 19%; stability = 47 ms; PARAD ON.
Therapy: VF = shock; VT = antitachycardia pacing and cardioversion.

Bradycardia settings
Mode: DDD 60–120 bpm.
Mode switch = ON.
AV = 188 ms.

Electrogram interpretation

1. *Assessment of the onset of the tachyarrhythmia triggering the device*: the first VV interval in the tachycardia detection zone triggering the device is not available in the electrogram.

2. *Comparison between atrial and ventricular rate*: rate branch VV > AA.
3. *Description of the atrial rhythm*: the wide-band electrogram shows small deflections, which represent the atrial activity (arrows in the figure below). The marker channel and the numerical annotations on the device activity channel confirm the atrial cycle length of 344 ms. The device activity channel also shows a pattern of four consecutive atrial activations followed by a "pause" of 688 ms. The pause in atrial activation can be explained by the presence of ventriculoatrial crossblanking of the device. The morphology of the atrial activity is consistent. The atrial rhythm demonstrates either sinus or atrial tachycardia.

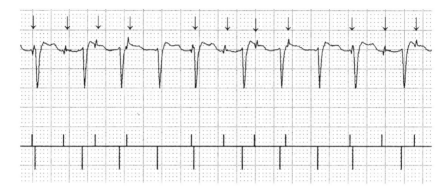

FIGURE 6.14b.

4. *Characteristics of the ventricular electrogram during the tachyarrhythmia*: the morphology of the ventricular activity is consistent during tachycardia. The tachycardia has a ventricular cycle length of ≈406 ms. The wide-band electrogram shows a pattern of four consecutive ventricular activations followed by a longer interval. This pattern is confirmed by the device activity channel.
5. *Atrioventricular relationship*: The atrioventricular conduction pattern can be assessed from the marker channel. During the tachycardia, a consistent pattern of the atrioventricular conduction can be assessed by a ladder diagram (see further). Of the four consecutive atrial activations, the "first" atrial activity is blocked in the atrioventricular node. The next three atrial activations are conducted to the ventricular with a progressive increase in the atrioventricular conduction time. The "fifth" atrial activation coincides with the ventricular activation caused by the conducted "fourth" atrial activation. This pattern repeats itself as can be assessed in the original electrogram. (*See* Figure 6.14c)

Diagnosis: sinus or atrial tachycardia with atrioventricular Wenckebach conduction pattern. The p wave is hidden in the QRS complex, and is not

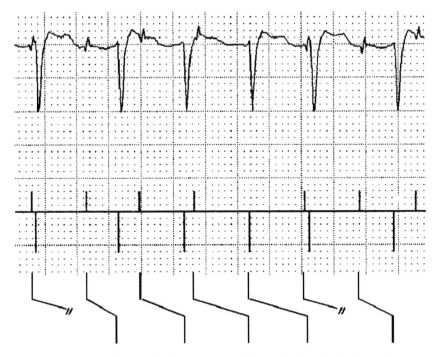

FIGURE 6.14c. From top to bottom: wide-band electrogram, device activity channel, and a ladder diagram.

displayed on the marker as it is within the post ventricular atrial blanking period.

Action: No further action

Case 15 ATP, Observed During Routine Control

Patient: 74-year-old female with ischemic heart disease, old inferoposterior wall myocardial infarction, left ventricular ejection fraction 0.19, documented paroxysmal atrial fibrillation.

Index arrhythmia: out-of-hospital cardiac arrest, ventricular fibrillation.

Complaint: no complaints were noted at follow-up, only events treated with antitachycardia pacing were obtained from the device's memory.

Electrogram

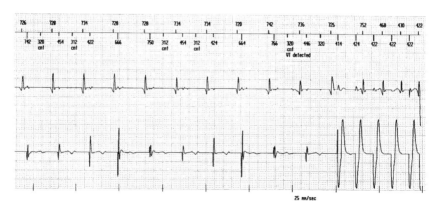

FIGURE 6.15a. From top to bottom: marker channel, atrial electrogram, and ventricular electrogram. Markers: CNT = count in tachycardia detection window.

ICD pulse generator: Phylax AV (Biotronik Inc, Berlin, Germany).

Tachycardia settings
Detection: VF = 300 ms; VT = 380 ms.
Discrimination: onset = 15%; stability = 40 ms; SMART ON.
Therapy: VF = shock; VT = antitachycardia pacing and cardioversion.

Bradycardia settings
Mode: DDD 60–120 bpm.
Mode switch = ON.
AV = 180 ms.

Electrogram interpretation

1. *Presence of tachyarrhythmia?*: No.
2. *Presence of high-frequency noise on isoelectric baseline?*: No.
3. *Description of the atrial rhythm*: the atrial electrogram shows both large as well as small deflections (upper electrogram). The small deflections represent far-field oversensing of the ventricular activity. The large deflection represents an atrial rhythm, cycle length ≈ 730 ms, with a consistent morphology. The atrial electrogram demonstrates sinus rhythm. The large deflections represent the baseline rhythm, cycle length ≈730 ms.
4. *Description of the ventricular electrogram*: the ventricular electrogram shows both large sharp deflections as well as small waves occurring at an interval of 320 ms after each sharp deflection. The sharp deflections represent the ventricular rhythm with a cycle length of ≈730 ms. The marker channel demonstrates more sensed ventricular activities than present on the ventricular electrogram. In Figure 6.15b, the sensed activities on the marker channel are related to ventricular electrogram. Sensed ventricular activity is displayed as "R" and "T" represents the T wave.

Diagnosis: T-wave oversensing caused inappropriate detection of ventricular tachycardia.

Action: programmation of specific sensing parameters to prevent T-wave oversensing. Automatic sensitivity control begins to adjust sensing threshold after a blanking period of 121 ms. This blanking period can be prolonged and/or the sensing threshold can be increased.

Relation between marker channel and ventricular electrogram

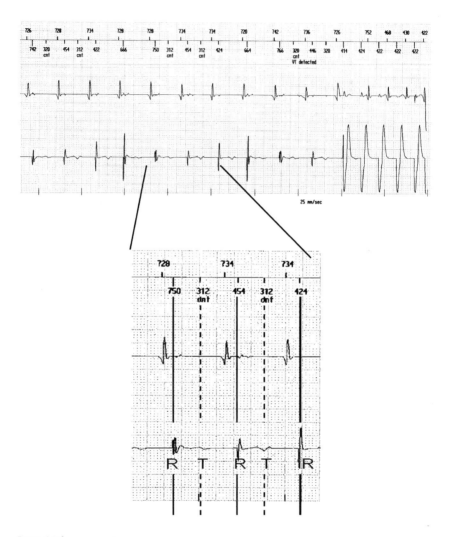

FIGURE 6.15b.

Case 16 Dizziness, Without Palpitations

Patient: 76-year-old male with coronary artery disease and preserved ventricular function.

Index arrhythmia: sustained monomorphic ventricular tachycardia, cycle length 300 ms.

Complaint: dizziness, shock while working in a boat. This strip precedes antitachycardia pacing and is the last episode before the checkup.

Electrogram

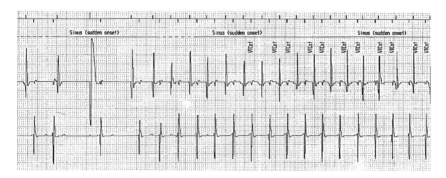

FIGURE 6.16a. From top to bottom: marker channel, atrial electrogram (in the former tracing also ventricular electrogram). VTCnt: counting of ventricular tachycardia. A ladder diagram is shown under the electrogram.

ICD pulse generator: Phylax AV (Biotronik, Erlangen Germany)

Tachycardia settings
Detection: VF = 280 ms; VT = 380 ms.
Discrimination: stability = 50 ms.
Therapy: VF = shock; VT = antitachycardia pacing.

Bradycardia settings
Mode: DDI 60 bpm.
AV = 250 ms.

Electrogram interpretation (*See* Figure 6.16b)

1. *Presence of tachycardia*: yes.
2. *Comparison between atrial and ventricular rate*: rate branch VV = AA.

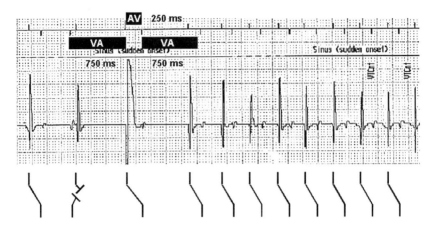

FIGURE 6.16b.

3. *Assessment of the onset of the tachyarrhythmia*: the marker channel illustrates how the second complex has a ventricular origin. It is followed by an atrial-paced sequence. This leads to a second pause, followed by the tachycardia with a supraventricular origin. It fulfills the criteria for sudden onset (from the second ventricular complex in the tachycardia on). The RR interval progressively becomes shorter than 400 ms, and the AV interval becomes longer.
4. *Description of the atrial rhythm*: the atrial activity on the marker channel shows a fast atrial rhythm with a cycle length around 400 ms. The atrial channel shows a far-field ventricular electrogram, has a stable morphology, and is comparable to the first complex. The atrial activity precedes the ventricular electrogram, except in the second complex, when the ventricular activity precedes the atrium (this is a VPB).
5. *Antitachycardia pacing (Figure 6.16c)*: does not affect this arrhythmia.

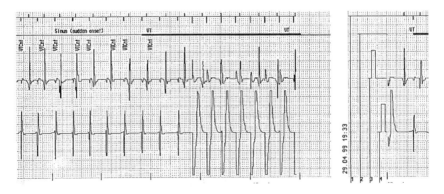

FIGURE 6.17b.
Diagnosis: sinus or atrial tachycardia with a cycle length < 380 ms.

Case 17 Self-terminating Tachycardia

Patient: 54-year-old female, heavy smoker with coronary artery disease, sequelae of anterior wall infarction, left ventricular ejection fraction of 29%, and congestive heart failure.

Index arrhythmia: short, fast monomorphic ventricular tachycardia, cycle length 300 ms, with syncope.

Complaint: shortness of breath.

Electrogram

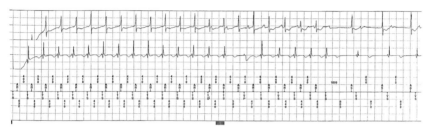

FIGURE 6.17a. From top to bottom: bipolar atrial electrogram, bipolar (near-field) ventricular electrogram, and marker channels. AP = atrial pace; AS = atrial sensing; AR = atrial refractory sense; VP = ventricular pacing; VS = ventricular sensing; TS = tachycardia sensing.

ICD pulse generator: GEM DR 7271 (Medtronic Inc, Minneapolis, MN, USA)

Tachycardia settings
Detection: VF = 320 ms; fast VT = 270 ms; VT = 400 ms.
Discrimination: stability = 50 ms.
Therapy: VF = shock; fast VT = antitachycardia pacing and shock; VT = monitor.

Bradycardia settings
Mode: DDD 40–115 bpm.
AV = 230 ms.

Electrogram interpretation (*See* Figure 6.17b)

1. *Presence of tachycardia*: yes.
2. *Comparison between atrial and ventricular rate*: rate branch VV = AA.

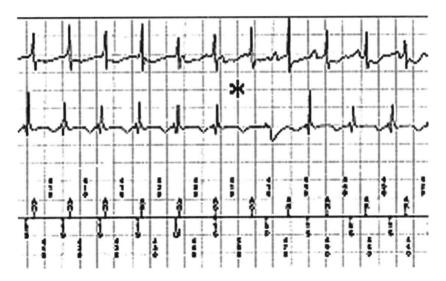

Figure 6.17b.

3. *Description of the atrial rhythm*: the atrial rhythm with CL of ≈410 ms is associated with a ventricular rhythm with the same CL. The atrial activity has the same, stable morphology as after termination, which excludes retrograde activation. The last atrial complex in the tachycardia precedes a ventricular complex.
4. *Assessment of the onset of the tachyarrhythmia*: is not shown in this rhythm strip, but was available (see below).
5. *Analysis of the atrioventricular (AV) relation*: brings the solution, as an atrial activity becomes non-conducted, and is followed after a pause (*) with ventricular pacing (VP). The atrial rhythm is unaltered by this event.
6. *Characteristics of the ventricular electrogram during the tachyarrhythmia*: the morphology of the ventricular activity is similar during tachycardia and after termination.

Marker channels of the onset

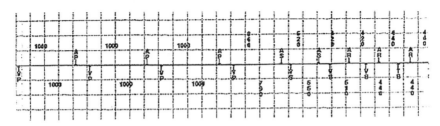

Figure 6.17c. AP = atrial pace; AS = atrial sensing; AR = atrial refractory sense; VP = ventricular pacing; VS = ventricular sensing; TS = tachycardia sensing. After atrial pacing, a gradually accelerating atrial activity precedes the ventricular activation, with slower AV conduction than during sequential pacing.

Diagnosis: atrial tachycardia with 1:1 conduction.

Case 18 An Unusual Association with Sudden Cardiac Death

Patient: 36-year-old lady with recurrent syncope, tongue biting, and seizures. Normal ECG with normal QT; K^+: 3.5 meq/l; frequent VPBs; non-sustained VT.

Index arrhythmia: collapse and resuscitation after polymorphic ventricular tachycardia in Neurology department.

Complaint: persistent dizziness.

Electrogram

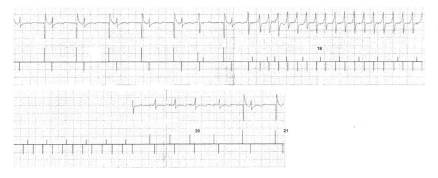

FIGURE 6.18a. From top to bottom: wide-band electrogram and marker channel.

ICD pulse generator: Alto DR 614 (ELA, Le Plessis, France).

Tachycardia settings
Detection: VF = 280 ms; VT = 345 ms.
Rate stability: 47 ms; onset 19%.
Therapy: VF = shock; VT = antitachycardia pacing and shock.

Bradycardia settings
Mode: DDI 70 bpm.
AV = 219 ms.

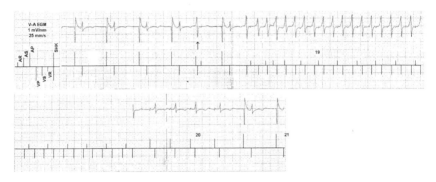

Figure 6.18b. Electrogram with calibration added. AP = atrial pace; AS = atrial sensing; AR = atrial refractory sense; VP = ventricular pacing; VS = ventricular sensing.

Electrogram interpretation (*See* Figure 6.18b)

1. *Tachyarrhythmia?* Yes.
2. *Comparison between atrial and ventricular rate*: rate branch VV < AA.
3. *Description of the atrial rhythm*: Initial atrial paced rhythm. Interrupted by a complex (arrow), when atrial and ventricular activity coincide (the electrogram suggests it is a VPB, with a wide QRS complex, and potentially a retrograde atrial activation). Further in the tracing, the atrial activity dissociates from the ventricular activity (clearly seen in the marker channel).
4. *Assessment of the onset of the tachyarrhythmia: judged from the electrogram*: the onset is a ventricular premature beat similar to the described one, again followed by a retrograde atrial activation.
5. *Characteristics of the ventricular electrogram during the tachyarrhythmia*: the morphology of the ventricular activity is not consistent during the ventricular tachycardia. The VA conduction pattern can be assessed from the marker channel and has a 2:1 pattern.

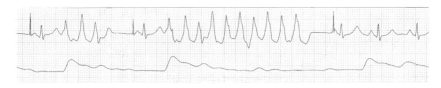

Figure 6.18c. Atrial pacing and non-sustained polymorphic tachycardia, initiated by VPB's with a reproducible QRS pattern, originating in the right ventricular outflow tract.

Diagnosis: non-sustained ventricular tachycardia.

Action: ablation of extrasystolic focus.

Case 19 A Fast, Almost Regular Rhythm

Patient: 74-year-old male with coronary artery disease and CABG; ejection fraction of 21%, paroxysmal atrial fibrillation; therapy with metoprolol.

Index arrhythmia: sustained monomorphic ventricular tachycardia, cycle length 360 ms.

Complaint: palpitations.

Electrogram

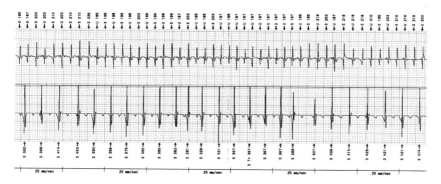

FIGURE 6.19a. From top to bottom: atrial electrogram, ventricular electrogram, and interval annotations.

ICD pulse generator: Tachos DR (Biotronik, Erlangen Germany)

Tachycardia settings
Detection: VF = 270 ms; VT = 400 ms.
Therapy: VF = shock; VT = antitachycardia pacing and cardioversion.

Bradycardia settings
Mode: DDD 50–120 bpm.
Mode switch = ON.
AV = 180 ms.

Electrogram interpretation (*See* Figure 6.19b)

1. *Comparison between atrial and ventricular rate*: rate branch VV < AA.
2. *Description of the atrial rhythm*: the atrial electrogram shows a fast, almost regular atrial rhythm with CL of 190–210 ms. The morphology is varying, but not to an extreme degree. The atrial rhythm can be classified as atrial flutter or tachycardia.

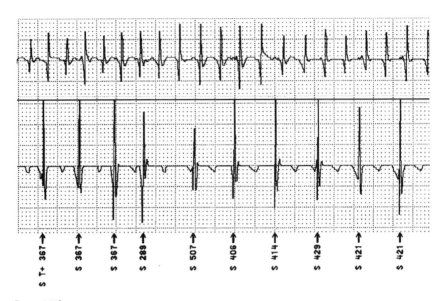

FIGURE **6.19b.**

3. *Assessment of the onset of the tachyarrhythmia*: not available here.
4. *Characteristics of the ventricular electrogram during the tachyarrhythmia*:
   the morphology of the ventricular activity is consistent during tachycardia,
   with one potentially different complex (after the pause of 507 ms in the
   second half). The atrioventricular relationship is compatible with atrial
   flutter and 2:1 conduction, which remains present also after the slowing of
   the atrial cycle to 210 ms. This explains the ventricular cycle length, initially
   about 380 ms, becoming 420 ms at the end of the rhythm strip.

Diagnosis: atrial flutter with predominantly 2:1 atrioventricular conduction.

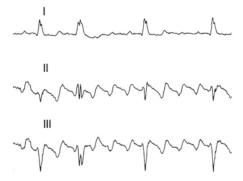

FIGURE **6.19c.** ECG taken at the time of consultation: typical atrial flutter, with 2:1 to 4:1 AV conduction (more
effect of the beta-blocker on the AV conduction).

Case 20 Unexplained High Frequency Potentials

Patient: 53-year-old male, with coronary artery disease (including CABG) and ventricular tachycardia since 13 years. Softball player.

Index arrhythmia: sustained ventricular tachycardia. ICD 2 years ago.

Complaint: Four shocks at home, without dizziness.

Electrogram (last shock – three continuous strips).

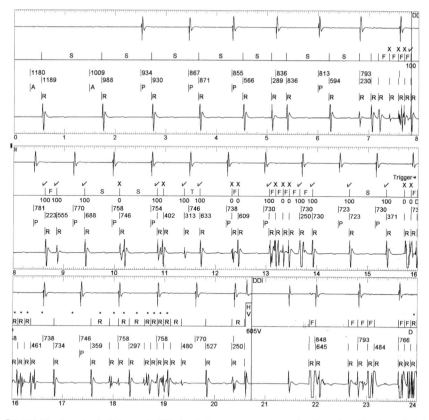

Figure 6.20a. From top to bottom: atrial bipolar electrogram; ventricular marker channel; atrial and ventricular intervals and markers; ventricular bipolar electrogram. A = atrial pace; F = ventricular fibrillation; P = atrial event; R = ventricular event; S = ventricular rhythm; T = ventricular tachycardia.

ICD pulse generator: Atlas DR V-240 (St Jude Medical).

Tachycardia settings
Detection: VF = 300 ms; VT = 430 ms.
Therapy: VF = shock; VT = antitachycardia pacing and cardioversion.

Bradycardia settings
Mode: DDI 50 bpm.
AV = 250 ms.

Electrogram interpretation

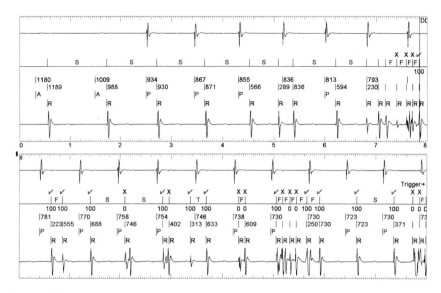

FIGURE **6.20b.**

1. *Tachycardia*: probably not.
2. *Comparison between atrial and ventricular rate*: VV < AA.
3. *Description of the atrial rhythm*: the atrial electrogram shows a regular, paced rhythm transitioning to an atrial rhythm which remains stable, and with the same morphology throughout the recording.
4. *Assessment of the onset of the tachyarrhythmia*: the onset is characterized by a premature beat in the ventricle, and several ventricular events with an extremely short coupling, sometimes with a high frequency.
5. *Characteristics of the ventricular electrogram during the tachyarrhythmia*: the morphology of the ventricular abnormal activity is different from the conducted beats. When using a caliper, it is possible to see that a normal QRS is seen after every atrial activity, with a normal AV interval. The events do not reset the atrial activity.
6. The atrioventricular relationship is unclear (see above).
7. The shock (HV) does not restore normality.

Surface ECG (V_4)

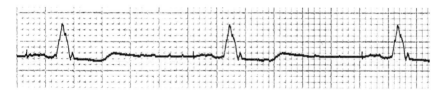

FIGURE 6.20c. Lead V4. Atrial pacing; no ventricular arrhythmia; tiny bumps/spikes are observed in the precordial leads; the relation with the intracardiac signals is not clear.

Suspected: noise at ventricular level, almost 2 years after implantation. Lead problem?

Actions

1. Measurement of the pacing and sensing characteristics – no changes vs before.
2. Shock delivery and measurement of shock lead impedance – no change of impedance after 0.1 J shock (40 ohm, as was previously known).
3. Local manipulation to provoke the abnormal electrograms (electrogram below).

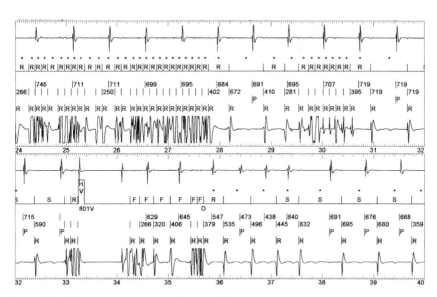

FIGURE 6.20d. This was easy – saturation of the amplifiers was evident (overflow to the atrial electrogram). The impedance did not change during this shock (39 ohm).

Conclusion: damage to the lead, not evident during assessment. Caused by action sports? Replacement of the lead.

Case 21 A Regular Tachycardia Triggering Device Therapy

Patient: 53-year-old male, coronary artery disease, inferior wall myocardial infarction, prior coronary artery bypass grafting, left ventricular ejection fraction 28%.

Index arrhythmia: sustained ventricular tachycardia, cycle length 400 ms.

Electrogram (obtained at the outpatient clinic).

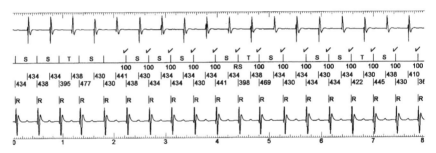

FIGURE 6.21a. From top to bottom: atrial electrogram, marker channel, and ventricular electrogram. Markers: ATP = antitachycardia pacing; D = detection; I = inhibtion by discriminators; P = atrial sense; R = ventricular sense; S = sense in the sinus window; T = sense in the tachycardia window; X = non-match; √ = match.

ICD pulse generator: Atlas DR V-240 (St Jude Medical, Sylmar, CA, USA).

Tachycardia settings
Detection: VF = 300 ms; VT = 430 ms.
Discrimination: onset = 16%; stability = 40 ms; morphology discrimination ON.
Therapy: VF = shock; VT = antitachycardia pacing and cardioversion.

Bradycardia settings
Mode: DDI 50 bpm.
AV = 250 ms.

Electrogram

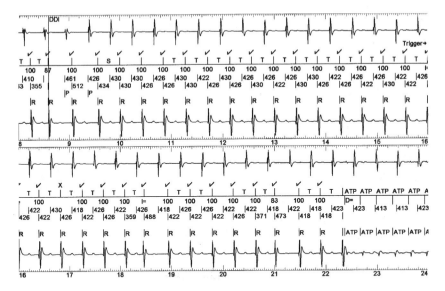

Figure 6.21b.

Interpretation

1. *Presence of tachyarrhythmia?*: Yes.
2. *Assessment of the onset of the tachyarrhythmia triggering the device*: the onset of the arrhythmia is not available in the electrogram.
3. *Comparison between atrial and ventricular rate*: rate branch VV = AA.
4. *Description of the atrial rhythm*: the atrial activity on the marker channel shows an atrial rhythm with an atrial cycle length ≈ 430 ms. The atrial electrogram shows a consistent morphology. The atrial rhythm is sinus tachycardia.
5. *Characteristics of the ventricular electrogram during the tachyarrhythmia*: the morphology of the ventricular activity is consistent in the electrogram, which is confirmed by the template match scores in the marker channel. The morphology of the ventricular electrogram is 100% (√) as compared to the template of the ventricular electrogram obtained during baseline rhythm. The atrioventricular conduction pattern can be assessed from the marker channel. During tachycardia, the marker channel demonstrates the presence of a consistent atrioventricular relationship. The ventricular rhythm has a cycle length of ≈ 430 ms, with a stability of ≈ 10 ms. Before deliverance of antitachycardia pacing, the ventricular electrogram shows two premature beats. The last premature beat causes a prolonged atrioventricular conduction in the next beat, which is confirmed by the device diagnostics (next page). The device classifies this as the presence of atrioventricular dissociation and subsequently therapy will be delivered.

Device diagnostics

TABLE 6.1.

Additional Information			
Initial Detection		Initial Diagnosis	
Initial Detection: Tach (141 bpm/425 ms)		Initial Diagnosis: Tach (142 bpm/420 ms)	
Result: SVT Criteria inhibited diagnosis.		Result: Diagnosis occurred; AV interval caused diagnosis of Tach.	
VT Diagnosis Criteria:	All	VT Diagnosis Criteria:	All
Rate Branch:		Rate Branch:	
Classification:	V = A Rate Branch	Classification:	V = A Rate Branch
AV interval:		AV interval:	
Programmed:	On, > 40 ms indicates AV dissociation	Programmed:	On, > 40 ms indicates AV dissociation
Measured Delta:	10 ms	Measured Delta:	50 ms
Morphology:			
Programmed:	On, ≥ 75% is a match, ≥ 5 of 8 matches indicate SVT		
Measured:			
Min Match Score:	100%		
Max Non-Match Score:	N/A		
No. Template Matches:	8 of 8 (SVT Indicated)		
Sudden Onset:			
Programmed:	On, < 16 % indicates SVT		
Measured Max Delta:	8 % (SVT Indicated)		

Interpretation

The left panel "Initial detection" shows that the discriminators "morphology" and "sudden onset" both indicated supraventricular tachycardia and therapy is inhibited. During ongoing detection, a change in atrioventricular conduction time triggered device therapy as can be observed in the right panel.

Diagnosis: inappropriately treated sinus tachycardia due to premature beats which caused a delay in atrioventricular conduction time.

Action: reprogrammation of the atrioventricular association time in the VV = AA rate branch.

Resynchronization Devices

Case 22 What to Do with this Complex Arrhythmia?

Patient: 59-year-old male with ischemic heart disease, left ventricular ejection fraction 0.31, congestive heart failure, and left bundle branch block (QRS width 132 ms).

History of paroxysmal atrial fibrillation, coronary artery bypass grafting. Index arrhythmia: sustained monomorphic ventricular tachycardia, cycle length 400 ms.

Complaint: palpitations.

Electrogram

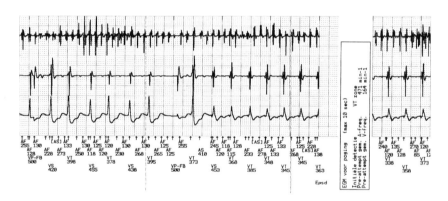

FIGURE 6.22a. From top to bottom: atrial electrogram, ventricular bipolar and shock electrogram. Markers: AF = atrial fibrillation window; AS = atrial sensing; VP-FB = ventricular pacing, fallback; VS = ventricular sensing; VT = ventricular tachycardia.

ICD pulse generator: Renewal H155 (Guidant Inc, St Paul, MN, USA).

Tachycardia settings
Detection: VF = 285 ms; VT = 415 ms.
Discrimination: onset = 16%; stability = 40 ms; V > A; Afib threshold < 300 ms.
Therapy: VF = shock; VT = antitachycardia pacing and cardioversion.

Bradycardia settings
Mode: DDD 70–120 bpm; mode switch = ON; AV = 70 ms.

Electrogram interpretation

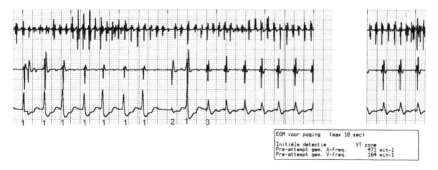

FIGURE **6.22b.** The insert annotates the electrogram, as being in the VT zone before the termination attempt, with the initial detection frequencies.

1. The first step in electrogram interpretation is the comparison between atrial and ventricular rate, which results in VV > AA rate branch.
2. The second step is a description of the atrial rhythm. The atrial electrogram shows a fast atrial rhythm with an atrial cycle length ≈ 125 ms with a changing atrial morphology. The atrial electrogram demonstrates atrial fibrillation.
3. The third step is the assessment of the onset of the tachyarrhythmia triggering device therapy. The ventricular and shock electrogram demonstrate normal conducted beats during atrial fibrillation, depicted as 1 in the electrogram. After a ventricular paced beat (VP-FB, fallback during mode switch, depicted as 2) and a normal conducted beat, a tachycardia is initiated (depicted as 3 in the electrogram).
4. Finally, we describe the characteristics of the ventricular electrogram during the tachycardia. The morphology of the ventricular and shock electrogram during tachycardia (3) changed as compared to the baseline rhythm (1). The tachycardia has a ventricular cycle length of ≈ 350 ms, with a stability of ≈ 20 ms. The AV relationship cannot be described during atrial fibrillation.

Diagnosis: ventricular tachycardia during atrial fibrillation.

Further actions: external cardioversion of persistent atrial fibrillation.

Case 23 Ineffective Antitachycardia Pacing

Patient: 59-year-old male with idiopathic dilated cardiomyopathy, left ventricular ejection fraction of 28%, congestive heart failure, and incomplete left bundle branch block (QRS width 100 ms).

Index arrhythmia: sustained monomorphic ventricular tachycardia, cycle length 200 ms.

Complaint: palpitations.

Electrogram

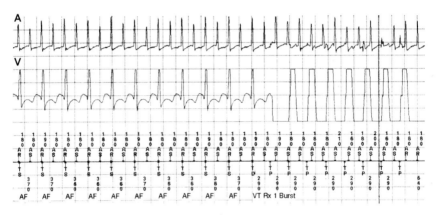

FIGURE 6.23a. From top to bottom: atrial electrogram – (A), ventricular electrogram – (V), and marker channel. Markers: AF = atrial fibrillation/flutter; AR = atrial refractory sense; AS = atrial sensing; TD| = tachycardia detected; TP = tachycardia pacing; TS = tachycardia sensing.

ICD pulse generator: InSync 7272 (Medtronic Inc, Minneapolis, MN, USA).

Tachycardia settings
Detection: VF = 250 ms; fast VT = 300 ms; VT = 400 ms.
Discrimination: stability = 40 ms; PR Logic ON.
Therapy: VF = shock; fast VT and VT = antitachycardia pacing and cardioversion.

Bradycardia settings
Mode: DDD 70–120 bpm; mode switch = ON; AV = 110 ms.

Electrogram interpretation

1. *Comparison between atrial and ventricular rate*: VV interval > AA interval.
2. *Description of the atrial rhythm*: the atrial activity on the marker channel shows a fast atrial rhythm with an atrial cycle length ≈180 ms. The atrial activity on the far-field electrogram shows a stable morphology with an alternans in amplitude. The atrial rhythm can be classified as atrial flutter or tachycardia.
3. *Assessment of the onset of the tachyarrhythmia triggering device therapy*: the marker channel demonstrates a stable ventricular rhythm with a consistent atrioventricular (AV) conduction pattern.
4. *Characteristics of the ventricular electrogram during the tachyarrhythmia*: the morphology of the ventricular activity is consistent during tachycardia. The atrioventricular conduction pattern can be assessed from the marker channel. During the tachycardia, the marker channel demonstrates a consistent atrioventricular relationship. The tachycardia has a ventricular cycle length of ≈360 ms, with a stability of ≈ 10 ms.

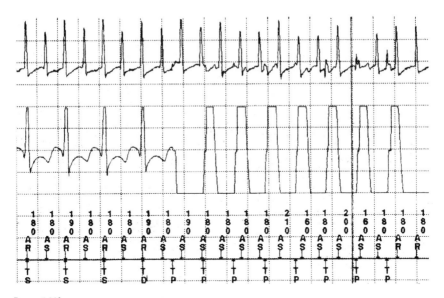

FIGURE 6.23b.

5. *Effect of therapy*: During ATP (TP), the atrial activity is unaffected with respect to rate and morphology.

Diagnosis: atrial flutter with 2:1 atrioventricular conduction.

Case 24 Back to the Ladder Diagram

Patient: 82-year-old female with dilated cardiomyopathy, congestive heart failure, left ventricular ejection fraction 0.30, left bundle branch block (QRS width 132 ms). History of paroxysmal atrial tachyarrhythmias.

Index arrhythmia: sustained monomorphic ventricular tachycardia, cycle length 320 ms.

Complaint: hospital admission after shock.

Electrogram (2 continuous strips).

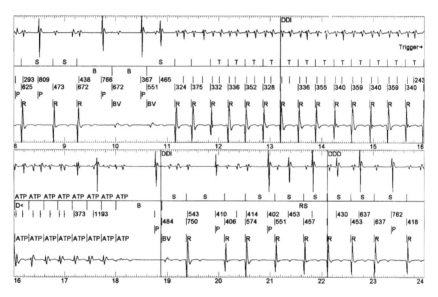

Figure 6.24a. From top to bottom: atrial electrogram, marker channel, and ventricular electrogram. Markers: B = bradycardia window; BV = biventricular pacing; P = atrial sense; R = ventricular sense; RS = return to sinus; T = ventricular tachycardia window.

ICD pulse generator: Atlas HF V-341 (St Jude Medical, Sylmar, CA, USA).

Tachycardia settings
Detection: VF = 300 ms; VT = 430 ms.
Discrimination: onset = 16%; stability = 40 ms.
Therapy: VF = shock; VT = antitachycardia pacing and cardioversion.

Bradycardia settings
Mode: DDD 60–100 bpm.
Mode switch = ON.
AV = 100 ms.

Electrogram interpretation

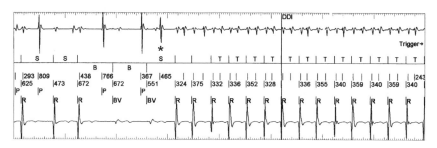

FIGURE 6.24b.

1. *Presence of tachyarrhythmia?*: Yes.
2. *Assessment of the onset of the tachyarrhythmia triggering the device*: a premature beat (*) initiates a fast tachyarrhythmia.
3. *Comparison between atrial and ventricular rate*: rate branch VV = AA.
4. *Description of the atrial rhythm*: the atrial electrogram shows large as well as small deflections. The small deflections represent far-field oversensing of the ventricular activity. The large deflection represents an atrial rhythm, cycle length ≈340 ms.
5. *Characteristics of the ventricular electrogram during the tachyarrhythmia*: the morphology of the ventricular activity is consistent in the electrogram. The morphology during tachycardia is similar to the morphology at baseline rhythm. The ventricular rhythm has a cycle length of ≈ 350 ms, with a stability of ≈ 10 ms. During tachycardia, the presence of a consistent atrioventricular relationship is observed (see ladder diagram below).
6. *Outcome of delivered device therapy*: ventricular antitachycardia pacing is effective.

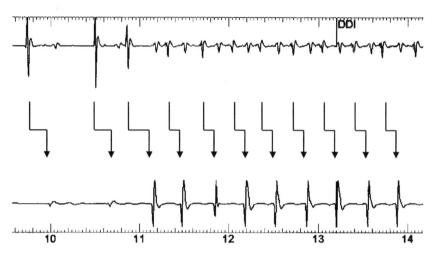

FIGURE 6.24c.

Ladder diagram during tachycardia (*See* Figure 6.24c)

Differential diagnosis tachycardia with 1:1 atrioventricular conduction

- The initiating event at the onset of tachycardia is identified at the atrial level;
- The morphology of the atrial activity during tachycardia is different as compared to baseline rhythm;
- The morphology of atrial premature beats is similar to the morphology of the atrial activity during tachycardia; and
- Presence of 1:1 antegrade atrioventricular conduction.

Diagnosis: inappropriate detection of atrial tachycardia with 1:1 atrioventricular conduction.

Action: activation of morphology discrimination; if possible, adjustment of atrial sensing to prevent far-field R-wave oversensing.

The first step in arrhythmia diagnosis by the device is the comparison of atrial and ventricular rates. The device misdiagnosed the tachycardia in the rate branch "VV > AA" due to far-field R-wave oversensing.

Case 25 Multiple Shocks During a Normal Heart Rate

Patient: 80-year-old male with ischemic heart disease, left ventricular ejection fraction 0.34, congestive heart failure, and left bundle branch block (QRS width 186 ms).

Index arrhythmia: sustained monomorphic ventricular tachycardias, cycle length 330 ms.

Complaint: recurrent high voltage shocks after ICD implantation.

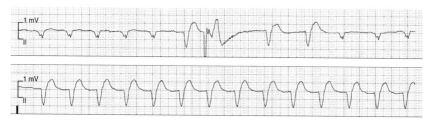

FIGURE 6.25a. Continuous ECG strip: Obtained during monitoring after ICD implantation. The patient experienced a delivered shock by the ICD.

ICD pulse generator: InSync 7272 (Medtronic Inc, Minneapolis, MN, USA).

Tachycardia settings
Detection: VF = 300 ms; fast VT via VF = 260 ms; VT = 370 ms.
Discrimination: stability = 40 ms; PR Logic ON.
Therapy: VF = shock; fast VT and VT = antitachycardia pacing and cardioversion.

Bradycardia settings
Mode: DDD 60–120 bpm.
Mode switch = ON.
AV = 150 ms.

Electrogram with interpretation (Two continuous strips). (*See* Figure 6.25b)

1. *Presence of tachyarrhythmia?*: No.
2. *Presence of high-frequency noise on isoelectric baseline?*: No.
3. *Comparison between atrial and ventricular rate*: unclear, ventricular markers suggest short VV intervals with no atrioventricular relation. If a laddergram would be drawn on part II of the electrogram it becomes clear that the ventricular depolarization is hidden in the artifact.

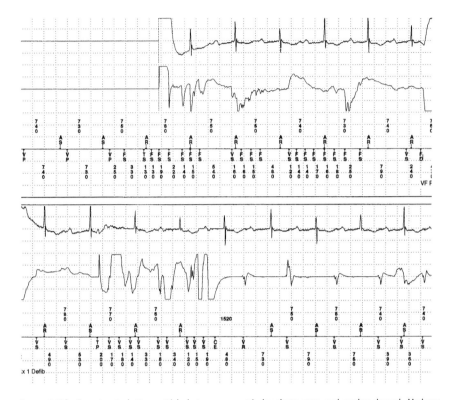

FIGURE 6.25b. From top to bottom: atrial electrogram, ventricular electrogram, and marker channel. Markers: AR = atrial refractory sense; AS = atrial sensing; CE = charge end; FD| = fibrillation detected; FS = fibrillation sensing; TS = tachycardia sensing; VP = ventricular pace; VR = ventricular refractory; VS = ventricular sense.

4. *Description of the atrial rhythm*: the atrial activity on the marker channel shows an atrial rhythm with an atrial cycle length ≈ 760 ms. The atrial activity on the atrial electrogram shows a stable morphology with changing amplitude, probably due to respiration. The atrial rhythm can be classified as sinus rhythm.
5. *Characteristics of the ventricular electrogram*: there is no distinctive morphology visible in the ventricular electrogram at the time of sensed ventricular activities. The ventricular electrogram shows intermittent baseline wander. Lead or connector problems resulted in intermittent saturation of the amplifier. (*See* Figure 6.25c)

Diagnosis: noise on the ventricular pace/sense lead, possibly due to loose connector.

Action: impedance measurement of the high voltage circuit and pace/sense circuit.

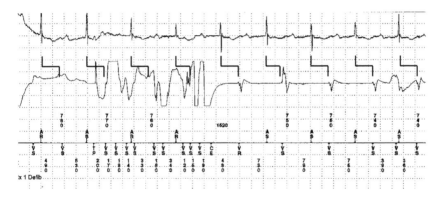

FIGURE 6.25c.

Lead or connector problems (header, adapter, or set-screw) may cause oversensing. The problem may be limited to the pace/sense lead and can be associated with postural changes. Abnormal pacing impedance is an indication of complete or partial interruption of the pace/sense circuit.

Impedance measurement demonstrated values of $>2000\,\mathrm{Ohm}$ for the pace/sense circuit. A loose set-screw of the pace/sense lead was observed during the surgical procedure.

Case 26 A Restrictive Cardiomyopathy with Wide Complex Tachycardia

Patient: 35-year-old female with old anterolateral myocardial wall infarction, left ventricular ejection fraction 0.35, restrictive dilated cardiomyopathy, QRS width 140 ms. Patient had a history of persistent atrial fibrillation.

Index arrhythmia: sustained monomorphic ventricular tachycardia, cycle length 270 ms.

Complaint: ICD delivered shocks.

Electrogram

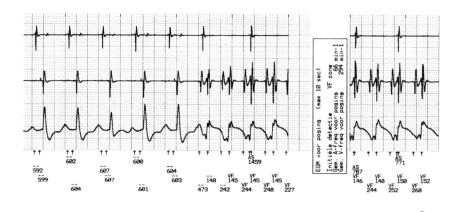

FIGURE 6.26a. From top to bottom: atrial, ventricular bipolar and shock electrogram. Marker annotations: AS = atrial sensing; Chrg = begin of charging; VF = fibrillation sensing; − = no annotation of events before detection of tachyarrhythmia.

ICD pulse generator: Contak CD (Guidant Inc, St Paul, MN, USA).

Tachycardia settings
Detection: VF = 300 ms; VT = 360 ms.
Discrimination: onset = 16%; stability = 40 ms; Afib threshold = 200/min;
V > A = ON.
Therapy: VF = shock; VT = antitachycardia pacing and cardioversion.

Bradycardia settings
Mode: DDD 60–120 bpm.

Mode switch = ON.
AV = 120 ms.

Electrogram interpretation

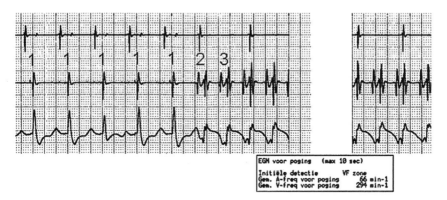

EGM voor poging   (max 10 sec)
Initiële detectie   VF zone
Gem. A-freq voor poging   66 min-1
Gem. V-freq voor poging   294 min-1

FIGURE 6.26b. The insert displays frequencies at initial detection.

1. *Presence of tachyarrhythmia?*: Yes.
2. *Assessment of the onset of the tachyarrhythmia triggering the device*: the ventricular and shock electrogram demonstrate biventricular pacing, depicted as 1 in the electrogram. After a ventricular premature beat (depicted as 2 in the electrogram), a tachyarrhythmia is initiated (depicted as 3 in the electrogram).
3. *Comparison between atrial and ventricular rate*: rate branch VV < AA.
4. *Description of the atrial rhythm*: the atrial electrogram shows large as well as small deflections. The small deflection represents far-field sensing of the ventricular activity. The large deflection represents an atrial rhythm with a cycle length ≈600 ms with a consistent morphology. The atrial electrogram demonstrates sinus tachycardia.
5. *Characteristics of the ventricular electrogram during the tachyarrhythmia*: the morphology of the ventricular and shock electrogram during tachycardia (3) changed as compared to the baseline rhythm (1). The tachycardia has a ventricular cycle length of ≈400 ms, with a stability of ≈10 ms. The atrial rate is not affected during the tachyarrhythmia, and there is no consistent atrioventricular relation. Each ventricular event during the tachyarrhythmia is sensed twice, which is confirmed by the marker annotations. As a result, a stable monomorphic ventricular tachycardia will be detected in the fibrillation detection window.

Diagnosis: ventricular double-counting during ventricular tachycardia.

Case 27 Cleaning and a High-voltage Shock

Patient: 55-year-old female, dilated cardiomyopathy, left ventricuar ejection fraction < 35%, heart failure, QRS width 166 ms, and a history of paroxysmal atrial fibrillation.

Index arrhythmia: non-sustained ventricular tachycardia.

Complaint: patient experienced a shock while cleaning.

Electrogram 1

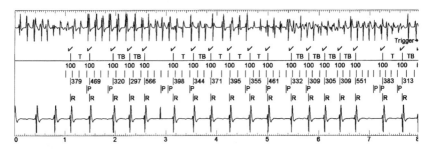

FIGURE 6.27a. From top to bottom: atrial electrogram, marker channel, and ventricular electrogram. Markers: I<= inhibition by discriminators; P = atrial sense; R = ventricular sense; T = sense in the ventricular tachycardia window; TB = sense in fast ventricular tachycardia window; √ = matched beat.

ICD pulse generator: Atlas HF V-341 (St Jude Medical, Sylmar, CA, USA).

Tachycardia settings
Detection: VF = 300 ms; FVT = 345 ms; VT = 400 ms.
Discrimination: onset = 16%; stability = 35 ms; morphology discrimination ON.
Therapy: VF = shock; FVT = antitachycardia pacing and cardioversion, VT = monitor.

Bradycardia settings
Mode: DDD 60–110 bpm.
Mode switch = ON.
AV = 90 ms.

Electrogram 2

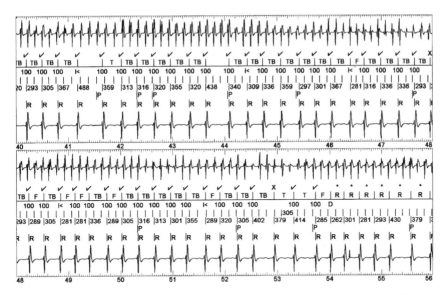

FIGURE 6.27b. From top to bottom: atrial electrogram, marker channel, and ventricular electrogram. Markers: D = detected; I<= inhibition by discriminators; F = sense in ventricular fibrillation window; P = atrial sense; R = ventricular sense; T = sense in the ventricular tachycardia window; TB = sense in fast ventricular tachycardia window; X = non-matched beat; √ = matched beat.

Interpretation

1. *Presence of tachyarrhythmia?*: Yes.
2. *Assessment of the onset of the tachyarrhythmia triggering the device*: in electrogram 1, the trigger is preceded by seven ventricular intervals annotated as being detected in the fast tachycardia detection window and five other intervals in the tachycardia window. The first detected ventricular interval in the tachycardia detection window is defined by the device as the onset of the tachyarrhythmia (V-V interval: 379 ms).
3. *Comparison between atrial and ventricular rate*: rate branch VV > AA.
4. *Description of the atrial rhythm*: the atrial electrogram shows a fast atrial rhythm with a cycle length ≈200 ms. The amplitude and the morphology of the atrial electrogram are constantly changing. The atrial electrogram demonstrates atrial fibrillation.
5. *Characteristics of the ventricular electrogram during the tachyarrhythmia*: the morphology of the ventricular activity is consistent in the electrogram. The marker channel shows 100% matching (√) of the ventricular electrogram during tachycardia with the ventricular electrogram obtained during baseline rhythm. The ventricular rhythm has a cycle length of ≈345 ms, with a stability of ≈150 ms (see tachycardia diagnostics below). Despite the unstable rhythm and no change in ventricular electrogram morphology, the patient experienced a shock delivered by the device.

Tachycardia diagnostics

TABLE 6.2.

Additional Information	
Initial Detection	Initial Diagnosis
Initial Detection: Tach B (173 bpm/345 ms)	Initial Diagnosis: Fib (206 bpm/290 ms)
Result: SVT Criteria inhibited diagnosis.	Result: Diagnosis occurred; SVT Criteria did not apply.

VT Diagnosis Criteria:	All
Rate Branch:	
Classification:	V < A Rate Branch
Morphology:	
Programmed:	On, ≥ 60% is a match, ≥ 5 of 8 matches indicate SVT
Measured:	
Min Match Score:	100%
Max Non-Match Score:	N/A
No. Template Matches:	8 of 8 (SVT Indicated)
Interval Stability:	
Programmed:	On, ≥ 35 ms indicates SVT (AVA Delta Passive, ≤ 60 ms indicates SVT)
Measured:	
Stability Delta:	150 ms (SVT Indicated)

Diagnosis: atrial fibrillation with a fast ventricular response. The discriminators "stability" and "morphology discrimination" both indicated atrial fibrillation.

The St Jude ICD compares the current interval with the average of the preceding intervals. Intervals are binned in a particular detection zone. When the current and the averaged intervals fall into two different detection zones, the faster interval is binned in the appropriate zone. This binning process is constant and the intervals are kept in their assigned detection zones. Based on the detection zone which reaches first the required number of intervals, the ICD will diagnose the tachyarrhythmia. In this case, the tachyarrhythmia was initially detected in the fast ventricular detection zone. The applicable discriminators inhibited the diagnosis of a ventricular tachyarrhythmia. After the initial diagnosis, the device will continue monitoring the rhythm (ongoing detection) to detect whether or not a ventricular tachyarrhythmia will develop. During this ongoing detection, intervals detected in the VF detection zone incremented the counter for VF detection despite appropriate diagnosis of atrial fibrillation.

Action

1. Increase the rate for detection of ventricular fibrillation.
2. Increase the number of intervals for detection of ventricular fibrillation.
3. Adjust pharmacological therapy to slow the ventricular rate.

Atrial Management Devices

Case 28 Wide Complex Tachycardia in a Lady with End-stage Cardiomyopathy

Patient: 45-year-old female with dilated cardiomyopathy; left ventricular ejection fraction 0.26, congestive heart failure, and left bundle branch block (QRS width 122 ms). History of atrial tachyarrhythmia.

Index arrhythmia: sustained monomorphic ventricular tachycardia, cycle length 420 ms.

Complaint: palpitations; VT suspected on the ward. Almost asymptomatic.

Electrogram

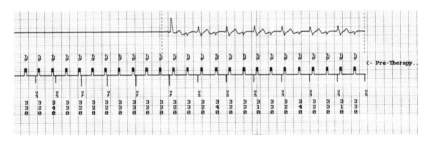

FIGURE 6.28a. From top to bottom: wide-band electrogram, markers, and marker channel. Markers: TD| = tachycardia sensing; VP = ventricular pace; VS = ventricular sense.

ICD pulse generator: Jewel AF 7250 (Medtronic Inc, Minneapolis, MN, USA).

Tachycardia settings
Detection: VF = 300 ms; VT = 460 ms.
Discrimination: stability = 40 ms; PR Logic ON.
Therapy: VF = shock; VT = antitachycardia pacing and cardioversion; AT = antitachycardia pacing.

Bradycardia settings
Mode: DDD 50–120 bpm.
Mode switch = ON.
AV = 180 ms.

Electrogram interpretation

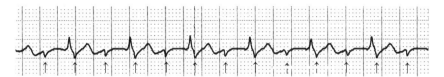

Figure 6.28b.

1. *Presence of tachyarrhythmia?*: Yes.
2. *Assessment of the onset of the tachyarrhythmia triggering the device*: the marker channel demonstrates a stable ventricular rhythm with a consistent atrioventricular (AV) conduction pattern.
3. *Comparison between atrial and ventricular rate*: rate branch VV > AA.
4. *Description of the atrial rhythm*: the atrial activity on the marker channel shows a fast atrial rhythm with an atrial cycle length ≈320 ms. The atrial activity on the far-field electrogram shows a stable morphology (↑). The atrial rhythm can either be an atrial tachycardia or an atrial flutter.
5. *Characteristics of the ventricular electrogram during the tachyarrhythmia*: the morphology of the ventricular activity is consistent in the electrogram. The ventricular rhythm has a cycle length of ≈650 ms, with a stability of ≈10 ms. During the stable ventricular rhythm, the marker channel demonstrates a consistent atrioventricular relationship with 2:1 atrioventricular conduction.
6. *Effect of therapy*: The marker channel shows atrial antitachycardia pacing (see below), which terminates the atrial tachyarrhythmia.

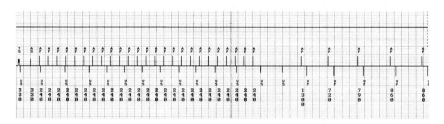

Figure 6.28c. From top to bottom: atrial and ventricular marker channels. Markers: AP = atrial pace; VP = ventricular pace; VS = ventricular sense.

Diagnosis: atrial tachycardia or atrial flutter.

Action: no further action.

Case 29 A Sudden Change in Ventricular Rate

Patient: 70-year-old male with ischemic heart disease, paroxysmal atrial fibrillation, coronary artery bypass grafting, left ventricular ejection fraction 39%.

Index arrhythmia: polymorphic sustained ventricular tachycardia.

Complaints: 6 weeks after ICD implantation multiple episodes treated with antitachycardia pacing.

Electrogram

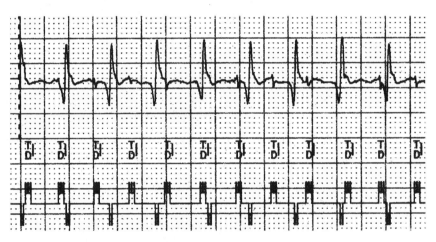

FIGURE 6.29a. From top to bottom: far-field electrogram (A-tip to V-ring), markers, and marker channel. Markers: TD| = tachycardia detected; TS = tachycardia sensing; VS = ventricular sensing.

ICD pulse generator: Jewel AF (Medtronic Inc, Minneapolis, MN, USA).

Tachycardia settings
Detection: VF = 320 ms; VT = 460 ms.
Discrimination: stability = 40 ms; PR Logic ON.
Therapy: VF = shock; VT = antitachycardia pacing and cardioversion.

Bradycardia settings
Mode: DDD 50–120 bpm.
Mode switch = ON.
AV = 150 ms.

Electrogram interpretation

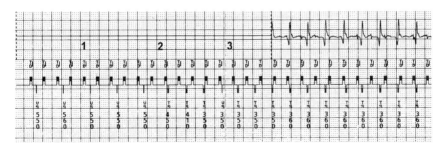

FIGURE 6.29b.

1. The first step in electrogram interpretation is the comparison between atrial and ventricular rate, which results in VV > AA branch.
2. The second step is a description of the atrial rhythm. The atrial activity on the marker channel shows a fast atrial rhythm with an atrial cycle length ≈ 280 ms. The atrial activity on the far-field electrogram shows a stable morphology. The atrial rhythm can either be an atrial tachycardia or an atrial flutter.
3. The third step is the assessment of the onset of the tachyarrhythmia triggering device therapy. The marker channel demonstrates a stable ventricular rhythm with a consistent atrioventricular (AV) conduction pattern, depicted as 1 in the electrogram. A premature beat (depicted as 2 in the electrogram) initiates a tachycardia (depicted as 3 in the electrogram).
4. Finally, we describe the ventricular electrogram morphology and the atrioventricular conduction pattern during the tachycardia. The morphology of the ventricular activity is consistent during tachycardia. However, the morphology cannot be compared to the baseline rhythm, as no electrogram is stored before arrhythmia onset. The atrioventricular conduction pattern can be assessed from the marker channel. The baseline rhythm (depicted as 1 in the electrogram) demonstrates a consistent atrioventricular conduction pattern. During the tachycardia, the marker channel demonstrates no consistent atrioventricular conduction pattern. The tachycardia has a ventricular cycle length of ≈ 360 ms, with a stability of ≈ 10 ms.

Diagnosis: ventricular tachycardia during atrial flutter or atrial tachycardia. The electrogram alone was not sufficient for the diagnosis.

Case 30 A Businessman Traveling to the Middle East

Patient: 60-year-old male, with paroxysmal atrial fibrillation who cardioverts himself with a patient activator, while traveling and buying carpets. Flecainide and bisoprolol.

Index arrhythmia: atrial fibrillation, atrial flutter.

Complaint: palpitations, failed shocks at home.

Electrogram

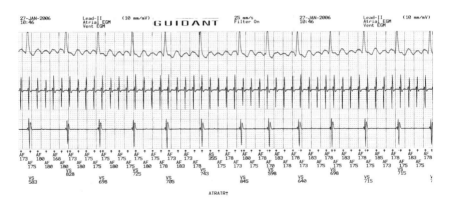

FIGURE 6.30a. From top to bottom: lead II, atrial and ventricular electrogram. AF = atrial fibrillation; VS = ventricular event.

ICD pulse generator: Vitality AVT (Guidant); coronary sinus shock lead.

Tachycardia settings
Detection: VF = 275 ms (15 sec); AT = 320 ms; AF = 240 ms.
Therapy: VF = shock; AT = antitachycardia pacing; AF = patient − controlled shock.

Bradycardia settings
Mode: DDD 60–140 bpm.
Mode switch = ON.
AV = 180 ms.

Electrogram interpretation

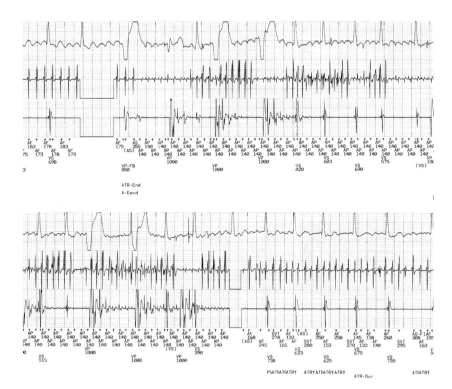

Figure 6.30b.

1. *Tachycardia*: yes. Very suggestive for atrial fibrillation in lead II.
2. *Comparison between atrial and ventricular rate*: VV > AA.
3. *Description of the atrial rhythm*: the atrial electrogram shows a very fast, regular atrial rhythm with CL of 180 ms. The morphology is constant. The atrial rhythm can be classified as atrial flutter.
4. *Assessment of the onset of the tachyarrhythmia*: not available here.
5. *Characteristics of the ventricular electrogram during the tachyarrhythmia*: only one QRS is shown in the initial part of this recording, the second electrogram is hidden by the onset of ATP. In the first recording, all ventricular electrograms are similar to each other.
6. The *atrioventricular relationship* is compatible with atrial flutter with a 4:1 relation.
7. *Effect of antitachycardia pacing*: degeneration to atrial fibrillation, with some wide QRS complexes, due to ventricular pacing.

Diagnosis: atrial flutter with 4:1 atrioventricular conduction. After ATP, atrial fibrillation becomes present. He will shock himself with the patient activator.

Case 31 Multiple Shocks on the Waiting List for Heart Transplantation

Patient: 43-year-old male, with coronary artery disease, heart failure NYHA class III, on the waiting list for heart transplantation. ICD at age 41, recent admission with exacerbation of heart failure, treated with diuretics. Discharged from hospital 2 weeks before the event.

Index arrhythmia: non-sustained ventricular tachycardia.

Complaint: six shocks, no palpitations, no chest pain.

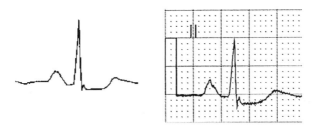

FIGURE 6.31a. Electrocardiogram (lead II): at previous control (left) and at admission (right). No new Q waves, nor ST elevations were seen.

ICD pulse generator: Marquis VR 7230 (Medtronic, Minneapolis).

Tachycardia settings
Detection: VF = 330 ms; FVT = 240 ms (via VF); VT = 360 ms.
Discrimination: onset = 88%; stability = 40 ms; wavelet ON, threshold 70%.
Therapy: VF = shock; FVT = antitachycardia pacing (burst), VT = monitor.

Bradycardia settings
Mode: VVI 40 bpm.

Electrocardiogram interpretation
The P wave has an amplitude of 2.5 mV and a width of 160 ms. This is similar compared to former tracings. The ST depression of 2 mm is now very prominent.

Initial tachogram

VT/VF Episode #3 Report

ID#	Date/Time	Type	V. Cycle	Last Rx	Success	Duration
3	May 26 17:39:09	FVT	300 ms	FVT Rx 6	No	2.7 min

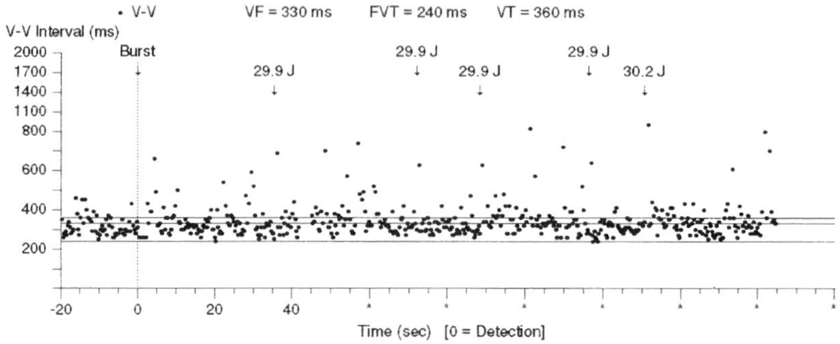

FIGURE 6.31b. The interval plot shows variable V-V intervals, several fall within the VT one and the normal zone; the majority lies within the VF zone. After burst pacing, five shocks are delivered.

In the second tachogram (not shown), the same arrhythmia is present, and three additional shocks are given, resulting in a slower irregular rhythm.

Last tachogram

VT/VF Episode #5 Report

ID#	Date/Time	Type	V. Cycle	Last Rx	Success	Duration
5	May 26 17:48:31	FVT	270 ms	FVT Rx 1	Yes	13 sec

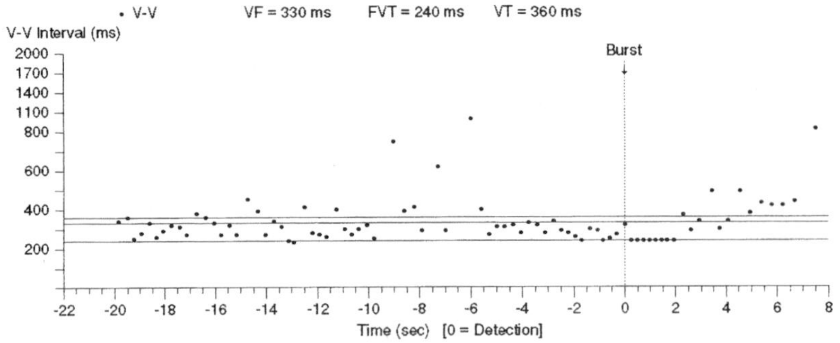

FIGURE 6.31c. A burst ATP episode converts the fast arrhythmia to a slower one. The electrogram of this last episode is shown below.

Electrogram

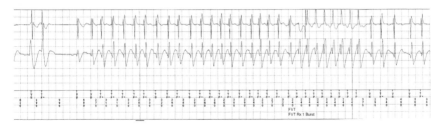

Figure 6.31d. From top to bottom: ventricular bipolar and wide-band electrogram, with marker channels. TF. = ventricular sense, fast ventricular tachycardia window; TP = pacing for tachycardia; TS = tachycardia sensing; VS = ventricular sense.

1. *Tachycardia*: present, highly irregular (cycle length 240–400 ms; bringing the rhythm in the FVT zone). FVT is confirmed.
2. *Assessment of the onset of the tachyarrhythmia*: the baseline rhythm is probably sinus rhythm, with atrial extrasystoles and a fast conducted atrial fibrillation.
3. *Characteristics of the ventricular electrogram during the tachyarrhythmia*: the morphology of the ventricular activity is similar during tachycardia, and during the complexes after ATP; before onset the complexes are somewhat different.
4. ATP (9 pulses) results in a slower rhythm, probably by making the AV-node refractory.

Diagnosis: atrial fibrillation resulting in multiple shocks. The patient had CK levels increasing to five times the normal value, and high Troponin T levels, making the diagnosis of non-ST segment elevation myocardial infarction likely. His potassium level was 3.5 meq/l.

Actions: reprogramming to single zone (VF, 230 bpm). An alternative would have been to create a VT zone with stability of 30 ms.

Case 32 An Episode of Atrial Bigeminy?

Patient: 70-year-old male with ischemic heart disease, old inferolateral wall myocardial infarction, left ventricular ejection fraction 0.27.

Index arrhythmia: sustained monomorphic ventricular tachycardia, cycle length 350 ms.

Complaint: Palpitations.

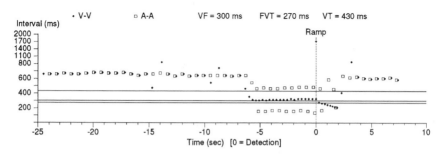

FIGURE 6.32a. ICD pulse generator: Marquis DR 7274 (Medtronic Inc, Minneapolis, MN, USA).

Tachycardia settings
Detection: VF = 300 ms; fast VT via VF = 270 ms; VT = 430 ms.
Discrimination: stability = 40 ms; PR Logic ON.
Therapy: VF = shock; fast VT and VT = antitachycardia pacing and cardioversion.

Bradycardia settings
Mode: DDD 70–120 bpm.
Mode switch = ON.
AV = 110 ms.

Electrogram (*See* Figure 6.32b)

Interpretation

1. *Interval plot*: the interval versus time plot demonstrates alternating AA intervals characterized by two rows of stable AA intervals (Figure 6.32a). The alternating AA intervals represent far-field oversensing of ventricular activity. The marker channel in the electrogram confirms the alternating AA intervals, ≈160 ms and ≈460 ms.
2. *Presence of tachyarrhythmia?*: Yes.

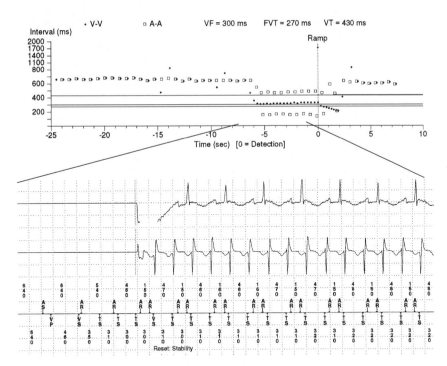

FIGURE 6.32b. From top to bottom: atrial electrogram, ventricular electrogram, and marker channel. Markers: AR = atrial refractory sense; AS = atrial sensing; TS = tachycardia sensing; VP = ventricular pace; VS = ventricular sense.

3. *Assessment of the onset of the tachyarrhythmia triggering the device*: the first VV interval in the tachycardia detection zone (indicated as VS in the marker channel) indicates the onset of the tachyarrhythmia. The subsequent VV intervals are in the tachycardia detection zone.
4. *Comparison between atrial and ventricular rate*: rate branch VV < AA.
5. *Description of the atrial rhythm*: the atrial electrogram shows large as well as small deflections. The small deflection represents far-field oversensing of the ventricular activity. The large deflection represents an atrial rhythm, cycle length ≈630 ms, with a consistent morphology. The atrial electrogram suggests sinus rhythm.
6. *Characteristics of the ventricular electrogram during the tachyarrhythmia*: the morphology of the ventricular activity is consistent during tachycardia. The tachycardia has a ventricular cycle length of ≈320 ms, with a stability of ≈10 ms. The atrioventricular conduction pattern can be assessed from the marker channel. During the tachycardia, the marker channel demonstrates a consistent atrioventricular relationship with 2:1 retrograde conduction. To exclude the presence of an accessory pathway, additional information is provided by observation of the atrial activity during ventricular antitachy-cardia pacing. During antitachycardia pacing the atrial rate is unaffected (electrogram below). The presence of an accessory pathway is excluded by this finding.

Electrogram at termination

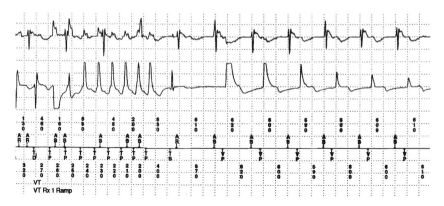

FIGURE 6.32c. From top to bottom: atrial electrogram, ventricular electrogram, and marker channel. Markers: AR = atrial refractory sense; AS = atrial sensing; TS = tachycardia sensing; TD| = tachycardia detected; TP = tachycardia pacing; VP = ventricular pace; VS = ventricular sense.

Diagnosis: appropriate detection of ventricular tachycardia with consistent far-field R-wave oversensing.

Action: no reprogrammation of the device.

Case 33 An Arrow on the Interval Plot

Patient: 60-year-old male with ischemic heart disease, coronary artery bypass grafting, left ventricular ejection fraction 0.17, QRS width 148 ms. History of paroxysmal atrial fibrillation.

Index arrhythmia: non-sustained ventricular tachycardias, inducible sustained ventricular tachycardia during electrophysiological testing.

Complaint: palpitations.

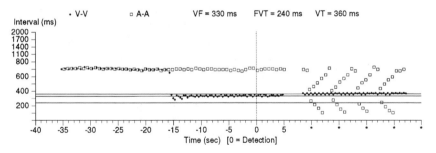

FIGURE 6.33a.

ICD pulse generator: Marquis DR 7274 (Medtronic Inc, Minneapolis, MN, USA).

Tachycardia settings
Detection: VF = 330 ms; fast VT via VF = 240 ms; VT = 360 ms.
Discrimination: stability = 30 ms; PR Logic ON.
Therapy: VF = shock; fast VT = antitachycardia pacing and cardioversion; VT = monitoring.

Bradycardia settings
Mode: DDD 70–120 bpm.
Mode switch = ON.
AV = 180 ms.

Electrogram interpretation

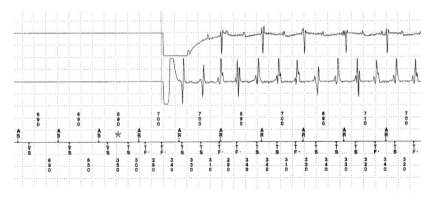

FIGURE 6.33b. From top to bottom: atrial electrogram, ventricular electrogram, and marker channel. Markers: AR = atrial refractory sense; AS = atrial sensing; TF. = ventricular sense, fast ventricular tachycardia window; TS = tachycardia sensing; VS = ventricular sense.

1. *Presence of tachyarrhythmia?*: Yes.
2. *Assessment of the onset of the tachyarrhythmia triggering the device*: the first VV interval in the tachycardia detection zone (*) indicates the onset of the tachyarrhythmia (upper electrogram). The subsequent VV intervals are in the ventricular tachycardia detection zone and fast ventricular tachycardia detection zone.
3. *Comparison between atrial and ventricular rate*: rate branch VV < AA.
4. *Description of the atrial rhythm*: the atrial electrogram shows large as well as small deflections. The small deflection represents far-field oversensing of the ventricular activity. The large deflection represents an atrial rhythm, cycle length ≈700 ms, with a consistent morphology. The atrial electrogram demonstrates sinus rhythm.
5. *Characteristics of the ventricular electrogram during the tachyarrhythmia*: the morphology of the ventricular activity is consistent during tachycardia. The atrioventricular conduction pattern can be assessed from the marker channel. During the tachycardia, the marker channel demonstrates absence of a consistent atrioventricular relationship. The tachycardia has a ventricular cycle length of ≈320 ms, with a stability of ≈20 ms.

Diagnosis: ventricular tachycardia, no therapy delivered because monitoring was programmed in the ventricular tachycardia detection zone.

Action: activation of antitachycardia pacing as therapy in the ventricular tachycardia detection zone.

Electrogram interpretation with tachogram (*See* Figure 6.33c)

Interval plot: the interval versus time plot demonstrates both an increase and a decrease in AA intervals, characterized by an "arrow" pattern. This

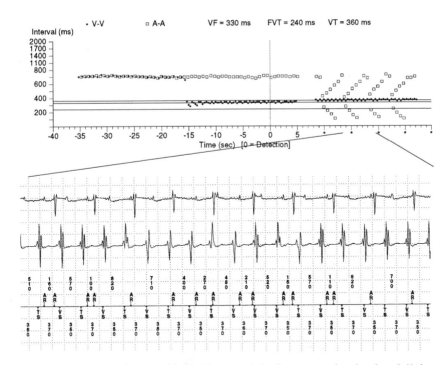

FIGURE 6.33c. From top to bottom: atrial electrogram, ventricular electrogram, and marker channel. Markers: AR = atrial refractory sense; TS = tachycardia sensing; VS = ventricular sense.

pattern is caused by the presence of far-field oversensing of ventricular activity during ventricular tachycardia with absence of a consistent atrioventricular conduction pattern. The increase is observed in AA intervals between atrial activity and far-field signal. The decrease is observed in AA intervals between far-field signal and atrial activity.

Case 34 Atrial Flutter with 2:1 Conduction?

Patient: 36-year-old male without structural heart disease, normal left ventricular function.

Index arrhythmia: out-of-hospital cardiac arrest, ventricular fibrillation.

Observation

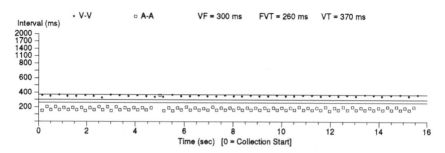

FIGURE 6.34a.

ICD pulse generator: Marquis DR 7274 (Medtronic Inc, Minneapolis, MN, USA).

Tachycardia settings
Detection: VF = 300 ms; fast VT = 260 ms; VT = 370 ms.
Discrimination: stability = 40 ms; PR Logic ON.
Therapy: VF = shock; fast VT = antitachycardia pacing and cardioversion; VT = monitoring zone.

Bradycardia settings
Mode: DDI 40 bpm; AV = 220 ms.

Electrogram interpretation (*See* Figure 6.34b)

1. *Interval plot*: the interval versus time plot demonstrates alternating AA intervals characterized by two rows of stable AA intervals. The alternating AA intervals represent far-field oversensing of ventricular activity. The marker channel in the electrogram confirms the alternating AA intervals, 160 ms and 190 ms.

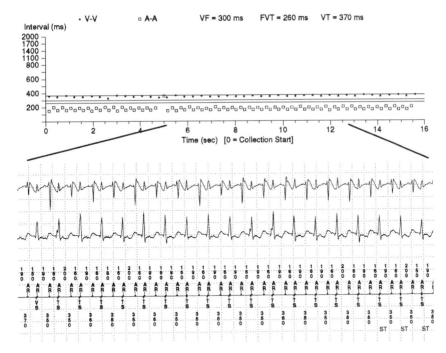

Figure 6.34b. From top to bottom: atrial electrogram, ventricular electrogram, and marker channel. Markers: AR = atrial refractory sense; ST = sinus tachycardia; TS = tachycardia sensing; VS = ventricular sense.

2. *Description of the atrial rhythm*: the atrial electrogram shows large as well as small deflections. The small deflection represents far-field oversensing of the ventricular activity. The large deflection represents an atrial rhythm, cycle length ≈360 ms, with a consistent morphology. The atrial electrogram demonstrates sinus tachycardia.

3. *Comparison between atrial and ventricular rate*: rate branch VV = AA.

4. *Assessment of the onset of the tachyarrhythmia triggering the device*: the first VV interval in the tachycardia detection zone (depicted as 1 in the electrogram) indicates the onset of the tachyarrhythmia. The subsequent VV intervals are in the tachycardia detection zone and when the programmed number of intervals for tachycardia detection (NID = 16) is reached, the annotation is ST (see marker channel).

5. *Characteristics of the ventricular electrogram during the tachyarrhythmia*: the morphology of the ventricular activity is consistent during tachycardia. The atrioventricular conduction pattern can be assessed from the marker channel. During the tachycardia, the marker channel demonstrates a consistent atrioventricular relationship, ≈160 ms. The tachycardia has a ventricular cycle length of ≈360 ms, with a stability of ≈10 ms.

Diagnosis: appropriate detection of sinus tachycardia with consistent far-field R-wave oversensing.

Action: no reprogrammation of the device. The consistent far-field R-wave oversensing is used by PR Logic in Medtronic dual-chamber ICDs to withheld device therapy during sinustachycardia. In case of consistent far-field R-wave sensing, it is recommended to activate the feature "other 1:1 SVTs" in PR Logic.

Case 35 Intermittent Atrial Tachycardia?

Patient: 36-year-old male without structural heart disease, normal left ventricular function.

Index arrhythmia: out-of-hospital cardiac arrest, ventricular fibrillation.

Observation

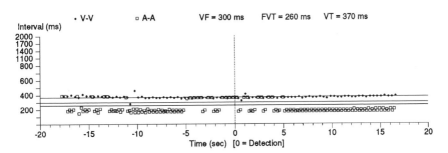

FIGURE 6.35a.

ICD pulse generator: Marquis DR 7274 (Medtronic Inc, Minneapolis, MN, USA).

Tachycardia settings
Detection: VF = 300 ms; fast VT = 260 ms; VT = 370 ms.
Discrimination: stability = 40 ms; PR Logic ON.
Therapy: VF = shock; fast VT = antitachycardia pacing and cardioversion; VT = monitoring zone.

Bradycardia settings
Mode: DDI 40 bpm.
AV = 220 ms.

Electrogram interpretation (*See* Figure 6.35b)

1. *Interval plot*: the interval versus time plot demonstrates intermittent periods of alternating AA intervals characterized by two rows of stable AA intervals. The alternating AA intervals represent far-field oversensing of ventricular activity, which is confirmed by the marker channel in the electrogram, 170 ms and 190 ms.
2. *Presence of tachyarrhythmia?*: Yes.

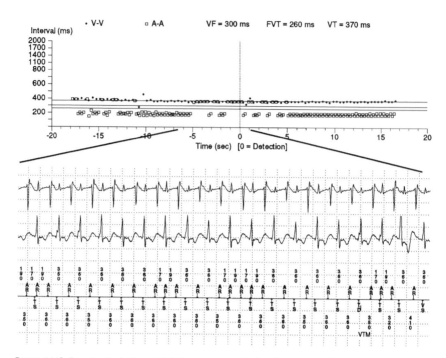

FIGURE 6.35b From top to bottom: atrial electrogram, ventricular electrogram, and marker channel. Markers: AR = atrial refractory sense; TD | = tachycardia detected; TS = tachycardia sensing; VS = ventricular sense; VTM = ventricular tachycardia monitoring.

3. *Comparison between atrial and ventricular rate*: rate branch VV = AA.
4. *Assessment of the onset of the tachyarrhythmia triggering the device*: the first VV interval in the tachycardia detection zone triggering the device is not available in the electrogram.
5. *Description of the atrial rhythm*: the atrial electrogram shows large as well as small deflections. The small deflection represents far-field oversensing of the ventricular activity. The large deflection represents an atrial rhythm, cycle length ≈360 ms, with a consistent morphology. The atrial electrogram demonstrates sinus tachycardia.
6. *Characteristics of the ventricular electrogram during the tachyarrhythmia*: the morphology of the ventricular activity is consistent during tachycardia. The atrioventricular conduction pattern can be assessed from the marker channel. During the tachycardia, the marker channel demonstrates a consistent atrioventricular relationship, ≈170 ms. The tachycardia has a ventricular cycle length of ≈360 ms, with a stability of ≈10 ms.
7. *Assessment of satisfied detection criteria*: the marker channel shows the annotation TD, which represents a satisfied tachycardia counter (16 consecutive intervals in the tachycardia detection zone, TS intervals). The far-field R-wave oversensing was not frequent enough during sinus tachycardia to withhold ventricular tachycardia detection. No therapy was delivered as the

tachycardia detection zone was programmed in a monitoring mode, which is represented by VTM in the marker channel.

Diagnosis: classification of sinus tachycardia as ventricular tachycardia due to intermittent far-field R-wave oversensing.

Action: reprogrammation of the device. In order to avoid arrhythmia misclassification due to intermittent far-field R-wave oversensing, the atrial sensitivity should be adjusted either to have consistent far-field R-wave oversensing or to eliminate completely far-field R-wave oversensing. If adjusting the atrial sensitivity is not satisfactory, the feature "other 1:1 SVTs" in PR Logic should be programmed OFF. The consistent far-field R-wave oversensing is used by PR Logic in Medtronic dual-chamber ICDs to withheld device therapy during sinus tachycardia. In case of consistent far-field R-wave sensing, it is recommended to activate the feature "other 1:1 SVTs" in PR Logic.

Case 36 Wide-complex Tachycardia after Cardiac Surgery

Patient: 41-year-old male patient, dilated cardiomyopathy, left ventricular ejection fraction 20%, congestive heart failure, left ventricular assist device, artificial respiration.

Index arrhythmia: primary prevention for sudden cardiac death.

Observation: no treatment for ventricular tachycardia.

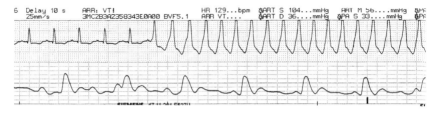

Figure 6.36a. Continuous ECG strip obtained during monitoring after cardiac surgery. The second tracing is the respiration.

ICD pulse generator: Entrust D154VRC (Medtronic Inc, Minneapolis, MN, USA).

Tachycardia settings
Detection: VF = 290 ms; FVT = 250 ms; VT = 370 ms.
Discrimination: stability = 30 ms; onset = 81%; wavelet ON, 70%.
Therapy: VF = shock; FVT and VT = antitachycardia pacing and cardioversion.

Bradycardia settings
Mode: VVI 40 bpm. (*See* Figure 6.36b)

Electrogram (*See* Figure 6.36c)

Interpretation

1. *Interval plot*: the interval versus time plot demonstrates a sudden decrease of ventricular intervals. The arrhythmia was classified as SVT despite the sudden onset of the tachyarrhythmia as shown in the interval plot.
2. *Presence of tachyarrhythmia?*: Yes.
3. *Assessment of the onset of the tachyarrhythmia triggering the device*: a premature beat (1) initiates a fast tachyarrhythmia (2).

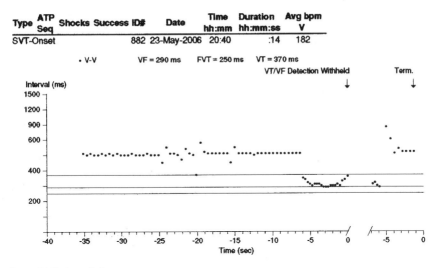

Type	ATP Seq	Shocks	Success	ID#	Date	Time hh:mm	Duration hh:mm:ss	Avg bpm V
SVT-Onset				882	23-May-2006	20:40	:14	182

FIGURE 6.36b. Interval plot

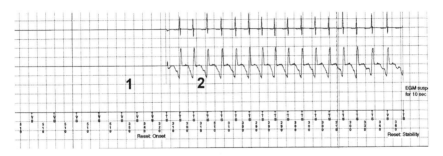

FIGURE 6.36c. From top to bottom: near-field ventricular electrogram, wide-band ventricular electrogram, and marker channel. Markers: TS = sense in ventricular tachycardia window; VS = ventricular sense.

4. *Characteristics of the ventricular electrogram during the tachyarrhythmia*: the morphology of the ventricular activity is consistent in both ventricular electrograms. The morphology cannot be compared to the baseline rhythm, as no electrogram was stored before arrhythmia onset. Additional information can be provided by the stored electrogram after arrhythmia termination (see figure 6.36d). The ventricular rhythm has a cycle length of ≈290 ms, with a stability of ≈10 ms.
5. *Characteristics of the ventricular electrogram after termination of the tachyarrhythmia*: the morphology after arrhythmia termination changed as compared to the morphology during the tachyarrhythmia.

Electrogram (*See* Figure 6.36d)

Diagnosis: fast monomorphic ventricular tachycardia with late coupled ventricular premature beat and slight irregularity. The device classified the

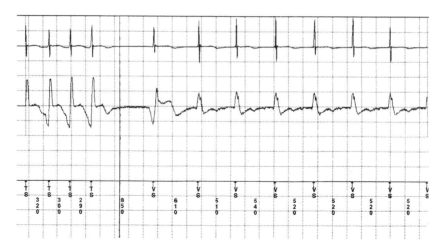

Figure 6.36d. Stored electrogram of spontaneous termination of the tachyarrhythmia. From top to bottom: near-field ventricular electrogram, wide-band ventricular electrogram, and marker channel. Markers: TS = sense in ventricular tachycardia window; VS = ventricular sense.

arrhythmia as SVT due to the calculation method of the onset and the stability of the tachycardia by the device. The calculated onset was gradual. The counting of tachycardia intervals was reset, put to "0", by the discriminator "stability" at the end of the rhythm strip.

Action: the discriminator "onset" was deactivated and the discriminator "stability" was increased from 30 ms to 50 ms to prevent underdetection of ventricular tachycardia.

Case 37 Transmitted Report of an Aborted High-voltage Shock

Patient: 84-year-old male patient with ischemic heart disease, chronic obstructive respiratory disease

Index arrhythmia: monomorphic sustained ventricular tachycardia, CL 330 ms.

Observation: Report transmitted by remote monitoring shows an aborted high-voltage shock.

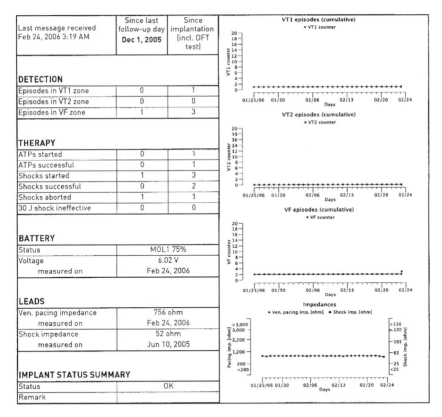

FIGURE 6.37a.

ICD pulse generator: Lexos VR-T (Biotronik Inc, Berlin, Germany). Epicardial lead system.

Tachycardia settings

Detection: VF = 300 ms; VT = 370 ms.

Discrimination: onset = 16%; stability = 40 ms.

Therapy: VF = shock; VT = antitachycardia pacing and cardioversion.

Bradycardia settings

Mode: VVI 50 bpm.

Electrogram

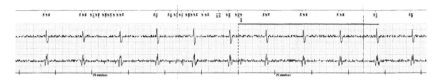

FIGURE 6.37b. Event which led to an aborted high-voltage shock. From top to bottom: marker channel, near-field ventricular electrogram, and wide-band ventricular electrogram. Markers: VF = sense in ventricular fibrillation window; VP = ventricular pace; VS = ventricular sense; VT-1 = sense in ventricular tachycardia window.

Interpretation

1. *Presence of tachyarrhythmia?*: No.
2. *Presence of high-frequency noise on isoelectric baseline?*: Yes.
3. *Description of the ventricular electrogram*: the morphology of the ventricular activity is consistent with a cycle length of ≈ 1000 ms and a stability of ≈ 10 ms. The marker channel demonstrates more sensed ventricular events than present on the ventricular electrogram. The wide-band ventricular electrogram shows both large complexes as well as small sharp deflections, which have no relation with the ventricular depolarization. The sharp deflections represent oversensing of signals which is confirmed by the interval plot.
4. *Interval plot*: the interval versus time plot shows a "rail track pattern," which represents oversensing.

Interval plot (*See* Figure 6.37c)

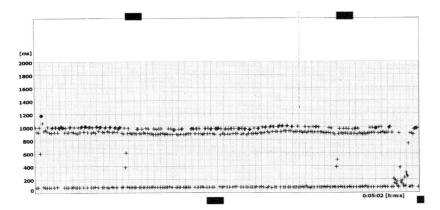

Figure 6.37c. Each "+" represents sensed ventricular activity.

Diagnosis: oversensing of signals.

Action

1. Local manupilation to provoke abnormal signals.
2. Measurement of lead impedance and shock system integrity.
3. Measurement of pacing and sensing characteristics.

Case 38 Slowing of the Heart Rhythm Followed by a Shock

Patient: 84-year-old male patient.

Index arrhythmia: monomorphic sustained ventricular tachycardia, CL 330 ms.

Complaint: patient experienced a shock.

Interval plot

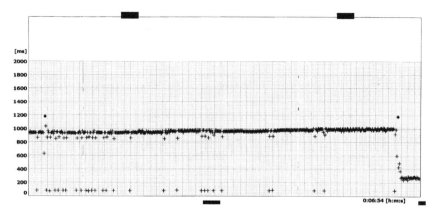

FIGURE 6.38a.

ICD pulse generator: Lexos VR-T (Biotronik Inc, Berlin, Germany). Epicardial lead system.

Tachycardia settings
Detection: VF = 300 ms; VT = 370 ms.
Discrimination: onset = 16%; stability = 40 ms.
Therapy: VF = shock; VT = antitachycardia pacing and cardioversion.

Bradycardia settings
Mode: VVI 50 bpm.

Electrogram (*See* Figure 6.38b)

Interpretation

1. *Presence of tachyarrhythmia?*: Yes.
2. *Assessment of the onset of the tachyarrhythmia triggering the device*: a premature beat (1) initiates a fast tachyarrhythmia (2).

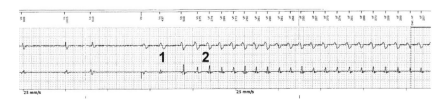

Figure 6.38b. From top to bottom: marker channel, near-field ventricular electrogram, and wide-band ventricular electrogram. Markers: VF = sense in ventricular fibrillation window; VP = ventricular pace; VS = ventricular sense.

3. *Characteristics of the ventricular electrogram during the tachyarrhythmia*: the morphology of the ventricular activity is consistent during tachycardia. The morphology of the ventricular electrogram changed as compared to the baseline rhythm, which is clearly in the wide-band ventricular electrogram. The tachycardia has a cycle length of ≈280 ms, with a stability of ≈10 ms.

Diagnosis: monomorphic ventricular tachycardia. The initiation is related to a paced beat, occurring after a pause.

Action: reprogrammation of the tachycardia detection zone to provide antitachycardia pacing as first therapy to terminate the arrhythmia. It is tempting to change the pacing mode to AAI, but this is evidently impossible.

Case 39 Wide-complex Tachycardia

Patient: 53-year-old male with ischemic heart disease, old myocardial infarction, left ventricular ejection fraction 30%, and QRS width 108 ms.

Index arrhythmia: non-sustained ventricular tachycardia, cycle length 330 ms.

Complaint: palpitations.

Interval plot

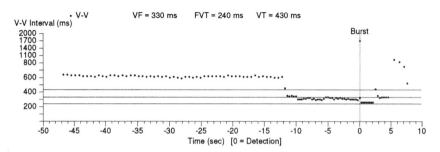

FIGURE 6.39a.

ICD pulse generator: Marquis VR 7250 (Medtronic Inc, Minneapolis, MN, USA).

Tachycardia settings
Detection: VF = 330 ms; FVT = 240 ms; VT = 430 ms.
Discrimination: onset = 88%; stability = 40 ms; wavelet = ON, 70%.
Therapy: VF = shock; FVT = antitachycardia pacing and cardioversion; VT = monitor.

Bradycardia settings
VVI: 40 bpm.

Electrogram (*See* Figure 6.39b)

Interpretation

1. *Presence of tachyarrhythmia?*: Yes.
2. *Assessment of the onset of the tachyarrhythmia triggering the device*: a premature beat (1) initiates a fast tachyarrhythmia (2).

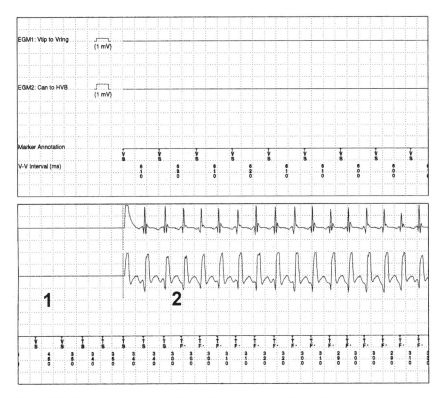

FIGURE 6.39b. From top to bottom: near-field ventricular electrogram, wide-band ventricular electrogram, and marker channel. Markers: TF = sense in fast ventricular tachycardia window; TS = sense in ventricular tachycardia window; VS = ventricular sense.

3. *Characteristics of the ventricular electrogram during the tachyarrhythmia*: the morphology of the ventricular activity is consistent during tachycardia. The morphology cannot be compared to the baseline rhythm, as no electrogram was stored before arrhythmia onset. Additional information can be provided by the stored electrogram after delivered device therapy (see below). Other additional information is given by the advanced diagnostics of this device, the comparison of the ventricular electrogram to the stored template of the baseline rhythm. In this figure, the template of the ventricular electrogram has changed from an "Rs" pattern during baseline, to a "qR" pattern during tachycardia. The tachycardia has a ventricular cycle length of ≈310 ms, with a stability of ≈10 ms.

4. *Characteristics of the ventricular electrogram after device therapy*: after antitachycardia pacing, the tachycardia continues with seven complexes and terminates spontaneously (see below). The morphology of the ventricular activity during sinus rhythm is different as compared with the morphology during tachycardia.

Stored electrogram of tachycardia termination

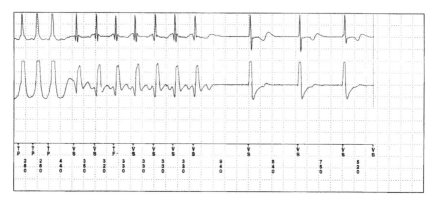

FIGURE 6.39c. From top to bottom: near-field ventricular electrogram, wide-band ventricular electrogram, and marker channel. Markers: TF = sense in fast ventricular tachycardia window; TP = antitachycardia pacing; VS = ventricular sense.

Wavelet analysis

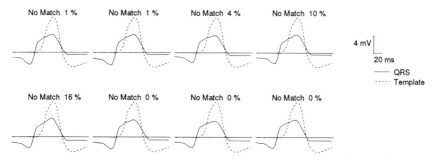

FIGURE 6.39d. Comparison between the ventricular electrogram during tachycardia (solid line) and the stored template of the baseline rhythm (dashed line). The template match between baseline rhythm and tachycardia is very poor, which classifies the tachyarrhythmia as ventricular.

Diagnosis: the tachycardia can either be of ventricular origin or atrial origin.

Action: no further action required.

Challenging Surface
Electrocardiograms

Case 40 Wide Complex Tachycardia

Patient: 60-year-old male with idiopathic dilated cardiomyopathy, congestive heart failure, left ventricular ejection fraction 28%, and QRS width 164 ms.

Index arrhythmia: sustained monomorphic ventricular tachycardia, cycle length 300 ms.

Complaint: palpitations.

Surface ECG

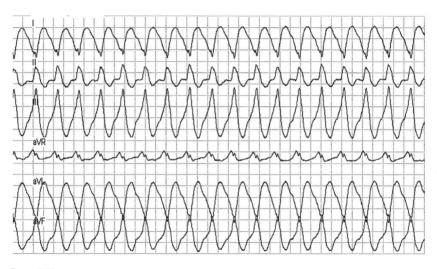

FIGURE 6.40a.

ICD pulse generator: Atlas VR V-199 (St Jude Medical, Sylmar, CA, USA).

Tachycardia settings
Detection: VF = 290 ms; fast VT = 360 ms; VT = 420 ms.
Discrimination: onset = 16%; stability = 40 ms; morphology ON.
Therapy: VF = shock; fast VT = antitachycardia pacing and cardioversion, and VT = antitachycardia pacing.

Bradycardia settings
Mode: VVI 60.

Interpretation of the surface ECG
Wide-complex tachycardia (QRS width 200 ms, cycle length 430 ms). Strictly

regular, monomorphic morphology, no atrial activity observed. The presumed diagnosis is ventricular tachycardia.

Electrogram during tachycardia

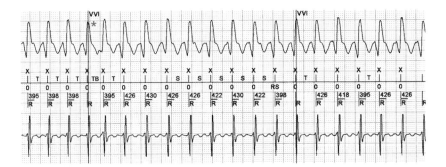

Figure 6.40b. From top to bottom: surface electrocardiogram (Lead II), marker channel, and ventricular electrogram. Markers: R = ventricular sense; RS = return to sinus; S = sinus sense; T = tachycardia sensing; TB = tachycardia sensing, tachycardia B window; X = no template match (morphology discrimination algorithm).

1. *Assessment of the onset of the tachyarrhythmia triggering the device*: the first VV interval in the tachycardia detection zone triggering the device is not available in the electrogram.
2. *Characteristics of the ventricular electrogram during the tachyarrhythmia*: the morphology of the ventricular activity is consistent during tachycardia. The surface ECG can be described as an "rSR complex" with a QRS width of 200 ms. The intracardiac ventricular electrogram shows an "rSRs" pattern. During tachycardia, the marker channel demonstrates a consistent template match score of 0%, as compared to the template obtained during sinus rhythm. The tachycardia has a ventricular cycle length of ≈415 ms, with a stability of ≈10 ms. The first VV intervals during tachycardia are within the detection zone for ventricular tachycardia (annotated as "T" in the marker channel). The marker "S" is related to VV intervals longer than the programmed tachycardia detection zone. The premature complex (*) with a coupling interval of 320 ms might be a fusion complex with the sinus beat, favoring the diagnosis of VT.
3. *Characteristics of the ventricular electrogram during sinus rhythm*: the final diagnosis based on the stored ventricular electrogram can be assessed when a stored electrogram displaying the rhythm after termination of the tachycardia (see figure 6.40c). The morphology of the ventricular activity during sinus rhythm is different as compared during tachycardia. The marker channel demonstrates a consistent template match score of 100% during sinus rhythm.

Electrogram during sinus rhythm

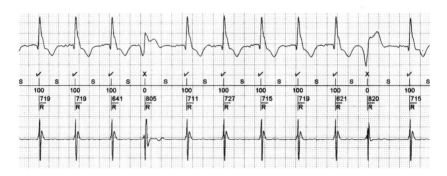

FIGURE 6.40c. From top to bottom: surface electrocardiogram (Lead II), marker channel, and ventricular electrogram. Markers: R = ventricular sense; S = sinus sense; X = no match with stored template (morphology discrimination algorithm); $\sqrt{}$ = template match.

Diagnosis: ventricular tachycardia, undetected.

Action: reprogrammation of the tachycardia detection zone; lowering the dosage of amiodarone.

Case 41 Acceleration of Polymorphic VT?

Patient: 76-year-old male with ischemic heart disease, old anterior wall myocardial infarction, prior coronary artery bypass grafting.

Index arrhythmia: recurrent ventricular tachycardia after out-of-hospital cardiac arrest.

Complaint: recurrent syncope.

Holter tracings

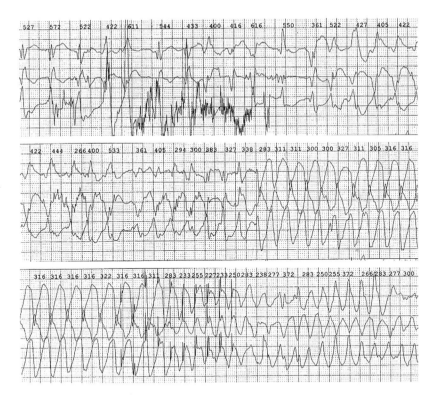

FIGURE 6.41a.

ICD pulse generator: Atlas VR V-199 (St Jude Medical, Sylmar, CA, USA).

Tachycardia settings

Detection: VF = 280 ms; VT = 430 ms.
Discrimination: onset = 16%; stability = 40 ms; morphology ON.
Therapy: VF = shock; VT = antitachycardia pacing and cardioversion.

Bradycardia settings

Mode: VVI 40 bpm.

Interpretation of the Holter registration

Holter recording shows wide QRS complex tachycardia which is treated with antitachycardia pacing, followed by acceleration.

Electrogram during tachycardia

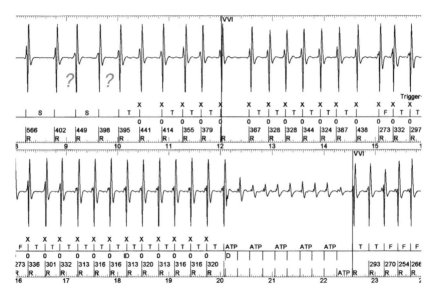

FIGURE 6.41b. From top to bottom: ventricular electrogram, marker channel, and device activity channel. Markers: ATP = antitachycardia pacing; D = fullfilled detection; F = ventricular fibrillation sensing; ID = inhibited diagnosis; R = ventricular sense; S = sinus sense; T = tachycardia sensing; X = no template match (morphology discrimination algorithm).

1. *Presence of tachyarrhythmia?*: Yes.
2. *Assessment of the onset of the tachyarrhythmia triggering the device*: the first VV interval in the tachycardia detection zone triggering the device is difficult to assess (? in the figure). In case of no clear onset of the tachyarrhythmia, the marker channel can give additional information. The VV intervals clearly recognized in the tachycardia detection zone are annotated as "T" in the marker channel.

3. *Characteristics of the ventricular electrogram during the tachyarrhythmia*: the morphology of the ventricular activity is consistent during tachycardia. The intracardiac ventricular electrogram shows an "rSRs" pattern. During tachycardia, the marker channel demonstrates a consistent template match score of 0%, as compared to the template obtained during sinus rhythm. Before antitachycardia pacing, the tachycardia has a ventricular cycle length of ≈315 ms, with a stability of ≈10 ms.

4. *Characteristics of the ventricular electrogram during sinus rhythm*: the final diagnosis based on the stored ventricular electrogram can be assessed with a stored electrogram displaying the rhythm after termination of the tachycardia (figure 6.41c). The morphology of the ventricular activity during sinus rhythm is different as compared during tachycardia. The marker channel demonstrates a consistent template match score of 100% during sinus rhythm.

Electrogram during sinus rhythm

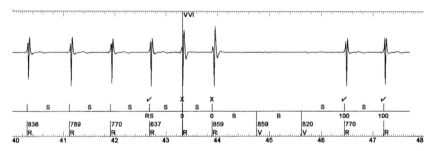

FIGURE 6.41c.

Diagnosis: slow ventricular tachycardia, appropriately detected by morphology discrimination. The antitachycardia pacing accelerated the tachycardia.

Action: adjustment of antitachycardia pacing.

Case 42 Pacing Induced Atrial Arrhythmia?

Patient: 45-year-old female with ischemic heart disease, left ventricular ejection fraction 0.26, congestive heart failure, and left bundle branch block (QRS width 122 ms). History of atrial tachyarrhythmia.

Index arrhythmia: sustained monomorphic ventricular tachycardia, cycle length 420 ms.

Complaint: hospital admission due to recurrent ventricular tachyarrhythmias.

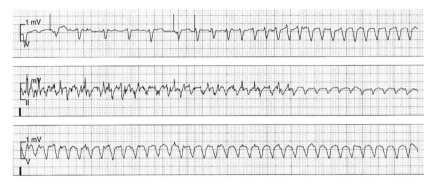

FIGURE 6.42a.

ICD pulse generator: Jewel AF 7250 (Medtronic Inc, Minneapolis, MN, USA).

Tachycardia settings
Detection: VF = 300 ms; VT = 440 ms.
Discrimination: stability = 40 ms; PR Logic ON.
Therapy: VF = shock; VT = antitachycardia pacing and cardioversion; AT = antitachycardia pacing.

Bradycardia settings
Mode: DDD 76–120 bpm.
Modeswitch = ON.
AV = 150 ms.

Electrogram interpretation

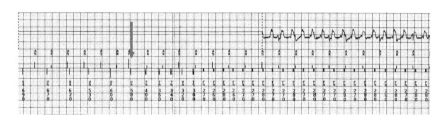

Figure 6.42b. From top to bottom: wide-band electrogram and marker channel. Markers: AP = atrial pacing; AR = atrial refractory sense; AS = atrial sensing; FS = fibrillation sensing; TS = tachycardia sensing; VP = ventricular pace; VS = ventricular sense.

1. *Presence of tachyarrhythmia?*: Yes.
2. *Assessment of the onset of the tachyarrhythmia triggering the device*: at the left site of the electrogram, the atrial activity on the marker channel shows an atrial rhythm with an atrial cycle length ≈440 ms. The atrioventricular conduction pattern during this atrial rhythm shows a Wenckbach pattern. An irregularity in the atrial sequence is observed, coinciding with a ventricular premature beat (arrow). This initiates a fast tachyarrhythmia.
3. *Comparison between atrial and ventricular rate*: rate branch VV < AA.
4. *Description of the atrial rhythm*: the atrial activity on the marker channel shows an atrial rhythm with an atrial cycle length ≈440 ms. The atrial activity on the far-field electrogram is by small deflections with a consistent morphology. The atrial rhythm can either be atrial tachycardia or sinus tachycardia. Regularity is resumed after the arrow, offering an argument to believe it was cross-sensing of the VPB.
5. *Characteristics of the ventricular electrogram during the tachyarrhythmia*: the morphology of the ventricular activity is consistent in the electrogram. The ventricular rhythm has a cycle length of ≈270 ms, with a stability of ≈10 ms. During the stable ventricular rhythm, the marker channel demonstrates absence of a consistent atrioventricular relationship. Additional information is provided by the marker channel after device therapy as no electrogram is available after therapy (see figure 6.42c). The marker channel demonstrates an atrial paced rhythm of 800 ms.

Diagnosis: double tachycardia, the patient has initially an atrial tachycardia with Wenckebach atrioventricular conduction pattern. During this atrial tachycardia, a ventricular premature beat induces a fast ventricular tachycardia. Pacing was atrial synchronous, in the ventricle.

Action: adjustment of antiarrhythmic drug treatment.

Marker channel after therapy

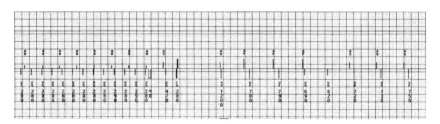

FIGURE 6.42c. From top to bottom: marker channel. Markers: AP = atrial pacing; AR = atrial refractory sense; AS = atrial sensing; CD = charge delivered; VP = ventricular pace; VS = ventricular sense.

Case 43 Incessant Tachycardia

Patient: 49-year-old female with ischemic heart disease, left ventricular ejection fraction 0.29, QRS width 170 ms, right bundle branch block.

Index arrhythmia: out-of-hospital cardiac arrest, ventricular fibrillation.

Complaint: shortness of breath, recurrent palpitations; admitted at hospital due to decompensation, incessant tachycardia (see ECG).

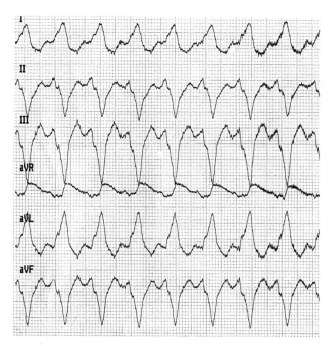

FIGURE 6.43a.

ICD pulse generator: Gem DR 7271 (Medtronic Inc, Minneapolis, MN, USA).

Tachycardia settings
Detection: VF = 280 ms; fast VT = 340 ms; VT = 440 ms.
Discrimination: stability = 40 ms; PR Logic ON.
Therapy: VF = shock; fast VT and VT = antitachycardia pacing and cardioversion.

Bradycardia settings
Mode: DDD 40–115 bpm.

Mode switch = ON.
AV = 230 ms.

Electrogram interpretation

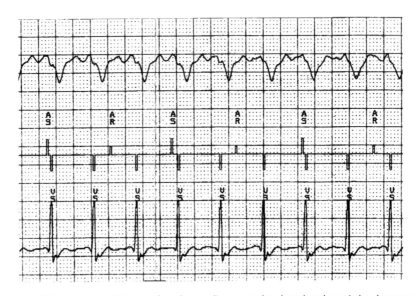

FIGURE 6.43b. From top to bottom: surface electrocardiogram, marker channel, and ventricular electrogram. Markers: AR = atrial refractory sense; AS = atrial sensing; VS = ventricular sense.

1. *Presence of tachyarrhythmia?*: Yes.
2. *Assessment of the onset of the tachyarrhythmia triggering the device*: not available in this electrogram.
3. *Comparison between atrial and ventricular rate*: rate branch VV < AA.
4. *Description of the atrial rhythm*: the atrial activity on the marker channel shows an atrial rhythm with an atrial cycle length ≈700 ms, without relation with the ventricular electrogram.
5. *Characteristics of the ventricular electrogram during the tachyarrhythmia*: the morphology of the ventricular activity is consistent in the electrogram. The ventricular rhythm has a cycle length of ≈480 ms, with a stability of ≈10 ms.

Diagnosis: slow ventricular tachycardia with absence of ventriculoatrial conduction.

Action: reprogrammation of the ventricular detection zone, hospitalization to diagnose the cause of the slow VT.

Case 44 Familial Sudden Death

Patient: 18-year-old boy whose father died suddenly at the age of 46, with a history of dilated cardiomyopathy. The boy showed exercise-related ventricular premature beats and short runs of polymorphic ventricular tachycardia, probably originating in the right ventricular outflow tract. After catheter ablation, an ICD was implanted.

Complaint: palpitations in spite of metoprolol.

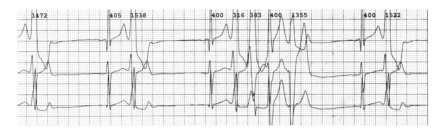

FIGURE 6.44a.

ICD pulse generator: Prizm DR 1861 (Guidant Inc, St Paul, MN, USA).

Tachycardia settings
Detection: VF = 250 ms; VT = 300 ms.
Discrimination: stability = 30 ms; onset = 16%; V > A = ON.
Therapy: VF = shock; VT = monitoring.

Bradycardia settings
Mode: DDI 40 bpm.
Modeswitch = OFF.
AV = 180 ms.

Interpretation of holter strip

The holter strip shows ventricular bigeminy with a short salvo of ventricular premature beats.

Electrogram interpretation (*See* Figure 6.44b)

1. *Presence of tachyarrhythmia?*: Yes.
2. *Assessment of the onset of the tachyarrhythmia triggering device detection*: the shock electrogram is helpful to assess the onset of the tachyarrhythmia. Fusion beats (*) initiate short tachyarrhythmias, falling in the VF detection zone.

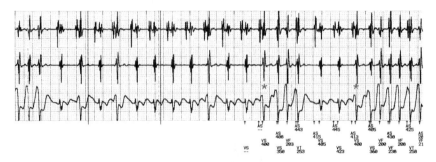

FIGURE 6.44b. From top to bottom: atrial electrogram, ventricular electrogram, shock electrogram, and markers. Markers: AS = atrial sensing; VF = fibrillation sense; VS = ventricular sense; VT = tachycardia sense.

3. *Comparison between atrial and ventricular rate*: rate branch VV < AA, based on the marker channel.
4. *Description of the atrial rhythm*: the atrial electrogram shows two deflections for every ventricular activity during baseline rhythm. The small deflection represents far-field oversensing of the ventricular activity. The large deflection represents an atrial rhythm, cycle length ≈ 425 ms. The atrial electrogram demonstrates sinus tachycardia with far-field R-wave oversensing.
5. *Characteristics of the ventricular electrogram during the tachyarrhythmia*: the morphology of the shock electrogram during tachycardia changed as compared to the baseline rhythm. The morphology of the ventricular activity is consistent in the shock electrogram during tachycardia. The ventricular rhythm has a cycle length of ≈245 ms, with a stability of ≈60 ms.

Diagnosis: sinus tachycardia with non-sustained ventricular tachyarrhythmias.

Action: adjustment of antiarrhythmic drug therapy. With regard to the far-field R-wave oversensing, no reprogrammation of the device is needed as the oversensing is captured in the blanking period after every sensed ventricular activity.

Case 45 TGA and Recurrent Atrial Flutter

Patient: 25-year-old male with surgically corrected transposition of the great arteries (Mustard operation), poor ventricular function, and recurrent atrial flutter.

Index arrhythmia: out-of-hospital cardiac arrest.

Problem: wide complex tachycardia after implantation detected on the monitor. This was not shocked.

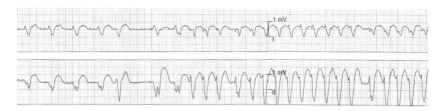

Figure 6.45a. Rhythm strip after implantation.

ICD pulse generator: Jewel AF 7250 (Medtronic Inc, Minneapolis, MN, USA).

Tachycardia settings
Detection: VF = 280 ms; VT = 340 ms.
Discrimination: stability = 30 ms; PR Logic ON.
Therapy: VF = shock; VT = monitoring.

Bradycardia settings
Mode: DDD 64–120 bpm.
Mode switch = ON.
AV = 150 ms.

Proposal: non-invasive induction with the ICD, with atrial stimulation.

Electrogram from EP study (*See* Figure 6.45b)

Electrogram during wide complex tachycardia (*See* Figure 6.45c)

Diagnosis: ventricular tachycardia. Undersensing of ventricular rhythm possible and demonstrated during ventricular fibrillation.

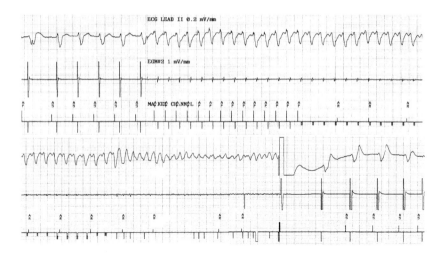

FIGURE 6.45b. From top to bottom: surface lead II, ventricular electrogram, and marker channel. Markers: AF = atrial fibrillation/flutter; AR = atrial refractory sense; AP = atrial pacing; AS = atrial sensing. After the first spike of a short burst of 15 atrial stimuli, the same arrhythmia as the clinical one is induced. AV dissociation is present. The ventricular electrogram shows a clearly reduced amplitude during tachycardia, but in the initial strip all events are recorded. The arrhythmia degenerates to ventricular fibrillation and is shocked, followed by atrial triggered pacing.

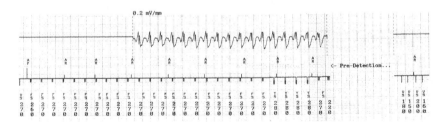

FIGURE 6.45c. Recording at 0.2 mV/mm from the ventricular electrogram. The amplitude is at least 1.8 mV. The QRS width is at least 0.16 ms, and the AV dissociation is clear. Markers: same on atrial level as above; TS = tachycardia sensed; FS = ventricular fibrillation sensed; VS = ventricular event sensing.

Action: reprogramming of ventricular sensitivity was impossible with this device, and remained at 0.3 mV.

Case 46 Wide Complex Tachycardia on Flecainide

Patient: 60-year-old male, with paroxysmal atrial fibrillation who cardioverts himself with a patient activator, while traveling. Flecainide and bisoprolol.

Index arrhythmia: atrial fibrillation, atrial flutter.

Complaint: palpitations, failed shocks at home.

Electrocardiogram: taken at emergency department (*See* Figure 6.46a)

ICD pulse generator: Prizm, AVT (Guidant); coronary sinus shock lead.

Tachycardia settings
Detection: VF = 275 ms (15 sec); AT = 320 ms; AF = 240 ms.
Therapy: VF = shock; AT = antitachycardia pacing; AF = patient-controlled shock.

Bradycardia settings
Mode: DDD 60–140 bpm.
Mode switch = ON.
AV = 180 ms.

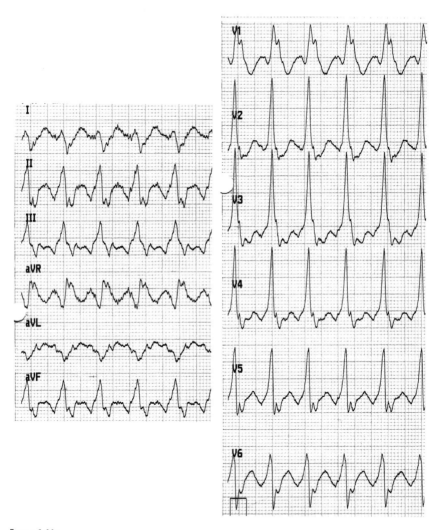

FIGURE 6.46a.

Electrogram with interpretation (*See* Figure 6.46b)

1. *Tachycardia*: yes.
2. *Comparison between atrial and ventricular rate*: VV > AA.
3. *Description of the atrial rhythm*: the atrial electrogram shows a fast, almost regular atrial rhythm with CL of 228 to 250 ms. The morphology is constant. The atrial rhythm can be classified as atrial flutter.
4. *Assessment of the onset of the tachyarrhythmia*: not available here.
5. *Characteristics of the ventricular electrogram during the tachyarrhythmia*: the morphology of the ventricular activity is consistent during tachycardia, with four complexes, every time after a longer cycle slightly different. This might be reflected by a wider S-wave in the surface electrogram.
6. The atrioventricular relationship is compatible with atrial flutter and 2:1 or 3:1 relation.

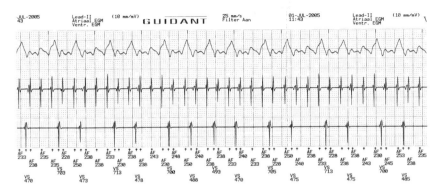

FIGURE 6.46b. From top to bottom: lead II, atrial and ventricular electrogram. AF = atrial fibrillation; VS = ventricular event.

Diagnosis: atrial flutter with aberrancy and predominantly 2:1 atrioventricular conduction.

Action: external shock, resulting in an atrial paced rhythm with narrow QRS complexes. A repeated cavo-tricuspid isthmus ablation is scheduled. (*See* Figure 6.46c)

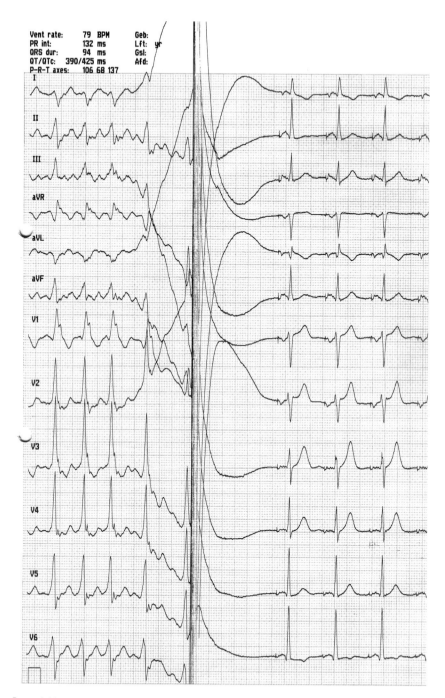

Vent rate: 79 BPM   Geb:
PR int: 132 ms   Lft: yr
QRS dur: 94 ms   Gsl:
QT/QTc: 390/425 ms   Afd:
P–R–T axes: 106 68 137

FIGURE 6.46c.

Case 47 Bradycardia Pacing and a High-voltage Shock

Patient: 57-year-old male, coronary artery disease, left ventricular ejection fraction 23%, QRS 160 ms, left bundle branch block.

Index arrhythmia: sustained monomorphic ventricular tachycardia.

Complaint: patient experienced a shock during hospitalization.

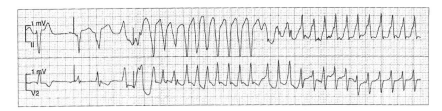

Figure 6.47a. Continuous ECG strip obtained during hospitalization for ventricular arrhythmias. The ECG strip shows a spike from the pacemaker during the vulnerable period of the ventricle (R-on-T), which is followed by a polymorphic ventricular tachycardia.

ICD pulse generator: Atlas HF V-341 (St Jude Medical, Sylmar, CA, USA).

Tachycardia settings
Detection: VF = 280 ms; VT = 410 ms.
Discrimination: onset = 16%; stability = 40 ms.
Therapy: VF = shock; VT = antitachycardia pacing and cardioversion.

Bradycardia settings
Mode: DDD 80–120 bpm.
Mode switch = ON.
AV = 250 ms.

Electrogram (*See* Figure 6.47b)

Interpretation

1. *Presence of tachyarrhythmia?:* Yes.
2. *Assessment of the onset of the tachyarrhythmia triggering the device:* a premature beat (*) inititates a fast tachyarrhythmia.
3. *Comparison between atrial and ventricular rate:* rate branch VV < AA. The electrogram shows only two intrinsic atrial complexes.

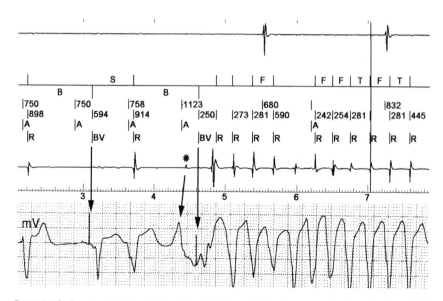

FIGURE 6.47b. From top to bottom: rhythm strip, with below atrial electrogram, marker channel, and ventricular electrogram. Markers: A = atrial pacing; B = bradycardia; BV = biventricular pacing; F = sense in fibrillation window; R = ventricular sense; T = sense in tachycardia window.

4. *Description of the atrial rhythm*: the atrial activity on the marker channel shows a paced atrial rhythm with a cycle length ≈750 ms; the amplitude of the paced atrial signal is very small. During the tachyarrhythmia, the atrial electrogram shows intrinsic atrial activity.
5. *Characteristics of the ventricular electrogram during the tachyarrhythmia*: the morphology of the ventricular activity is not consistent in the electrogram. The ventricular rhythm has a cycle length of ≈270 ms, with a stability of ≈10 ms. During the stable ventricular rhythm, the marker channel demonstrates absence of a consistent atrioventricular relationship.

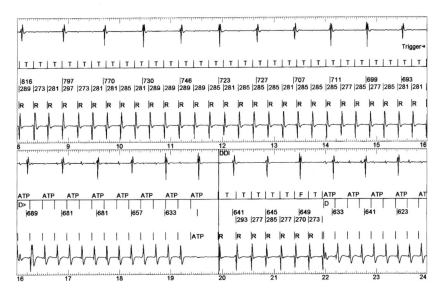

FIGURE 6.47c.

Diagnosis: at the onset of the arrhythmia, polymorphic ventricular tachycardia. This degenerates in a stable monomorphic ventricular tachycardia. ATP is given; it will accelerate the rhythm, so that finally a shock will be delivered. (*See* Figure 6.47c)

Case 48 Anticoagulation or Aspirin?

Patient: 60-year-old male, with no evidence of cardiac disease, and previous cardiac arrest 8 years ago. Aspirin, low dose sotalol because of paroxysmal atrial arrhythmia.

Index arrhythmia: ventricular fibrillation.

Complaint: palpitations, fatigue.

Electrocardiogram

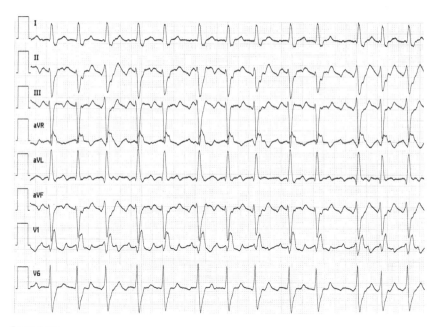

FIGURE 6.48a.

ICD pulse generator: Marquis DR 7274 (Medtronic).

Tachycardia settings
Detection: VF = 300 ms; FVT = 260 ms; VT = 360 ms.
Therapy: VF = shock; FVT = ATP + cardioversion; VT = monitor.
Discrimination: PR Logic = ON.

Bradycardia settings
Mode: DDI 35 bpm.
AVI = 200 ms.

Electrocardiogram interpretation

Typical counter-clockwise atrial flutter: dominant negative flutter waves inferiorly; positive waves in V_1 and negative waves in V_6.

Electrogram during checkup

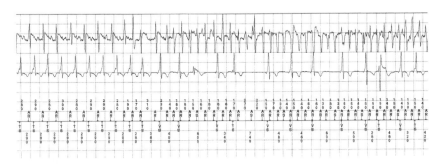

Figure 6.48b. From top to bottom: atrial and ventricular electrogram. Marker channels. AR = atrial refractory sense; AS = atrial event; TS: tachycardia; VS = ventricular event.

1. *Tachycardia*: yes. Initially very suggestive for atrial flutter with 1:1 conduction.
2. *Comparison between atrial and ventricular rate*: Initially, VV = AA, till the pattern changes at one-third of the rhythm strip.
3. *Description of the atrial rhythm*: the atrial electrogram shows initially a very fast, regular atrial rhythm with CL of 260 ms. The morphology is constant. The atrial rhythm can be classified as atrial flutter.
4. *Assessment of the onset of the tachyarrhythmia*: The onset is not displayed, but the change is initiated by a very short coupled atrial event (180 ms). This results in a very fast atrial rhythm, with a CL < 180 ms, and a much slower ventricular rate.
5. *Characteristics of the ventricular electrogram during the tachyarrhythmia*: all ventricular electrograms are similar to each other in the first part of the arrhythmia; two other morphologies are observed in the second part of the strip.
6. The *atrioventricular relationship* is compatible with atrial flutter with a 1:1 relation, degenerating in atrial fibrillation with slower AV conduction.

Diagnosis: atrial flutter with 1:1 atrioventricular conduction; atrial fibrillation becomes present.

Action: oral anticoagulation; scheduled for shock. Refused TEE guided approach.

Index

Printed in the United States of America.